'Since trauma is so painful to experience, people who have not suffered from it themselves tend to turn away from its victims and let them down. As a child and adolescent psychiatrist, I see it happening again and again. The book suggests that practice in confronting life's thorny and painful experiences — through mindfulness and self-compassion, for example — enhances our prospects of living as fully integrated people. The book has taught me new things about trauma and inspires me to learn more. I hope my colleagues in psychiatry will read it and ponder.'

Eva Henje Blom, associate professor, senior physician in child and adolescent psychiatry

'Live Now highlights the importance of specific knowledge in therapeutic work on severe trauma. It demonstrates that trauma processing must be given time and cannot be reduced to manualised instructions and predefined, short-term action programmes. Finally, the book emphasises the power of self-compassion and importance of victims learning to feel compassion for themselves — an ability whose value has recently gained attention in the context of not only trauma, but many other forms of mental suffering.'

Per Borgström, paediatrician, child psychiatrist, licensed and registered psychotherapist

'The book is about hope and healing just as much as pain and suffering. The stories testify that there is a way back to life despite deep traumatic wounds. It can take time and be arduous, but with gentle awareness and compassion the therapeutic healing begins. Live Now shows us that a meaningful and rewarding life is possible, after all.'

Joakim Gavazzeni, PhD in psychology

Life
whirls round
hither and thither
nudging and poking
inviting me to dance
romping and frolicking
coaxing out my chuckles
inflating my weak lungs
alluring and beckoning
with friendly insistence
awakening my senses
like a babbling brook
running untiringly
taking my hand
telling me to
come on
out

Clare James, after a poem in Swedish by Gabriella Luttrup

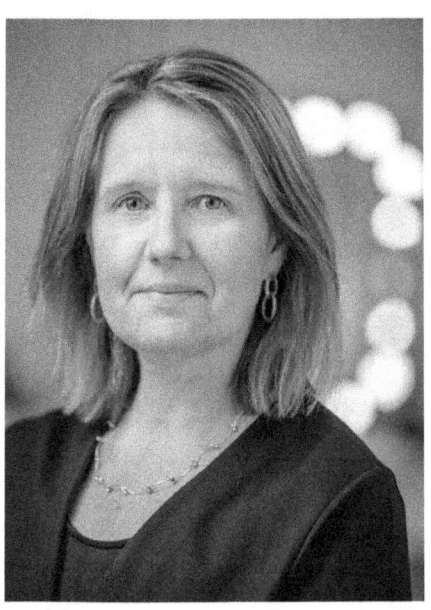

Annica Lilja Ljung is a licensed and registered psychotherapist with a degree in social work. For nearly all her working life, she has worked with traumatised people in child and adolescent psychiatric services, the former Crisis and Trauma Centre in Stockholm, adult psychiatric services and her own psychotherapy clinic. For many years, on courses, at conferences and with supervision by several world-leading teachers, she has specialised in trauma and dissociation.

info.annica@telia.com

www.traumacompassion.com

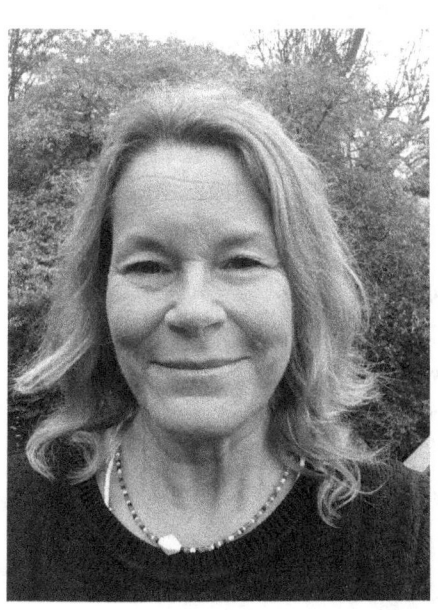

Christina Lejonöga, a freelance journalist, sees her writing as a form of socially critical social work in which she highlights victims who otherwise live in the shadows. She attaches great importance to retelling their stories in a manner as close to their own truth as could ever be possible. Over a prolonged period, she has interviewed the six main narrators in the book so as to truly give voice to their experiences.

christina.lejonoga@gmail.com

Voices on the book
Live Now: On Trauma and Dissociation

Immensely important reading for everyone working on trauma. All the theory feels vitally important. The authors write with warm hearts and great respect for the patients. Many people will learn to understand themselves — or their patients — better. I hope that Live Now will soon be found at every psychiatric and psychotherapeutic clinic, and on every study programme for psychologists, psychotherapists and doctors.

Elisabet Heigard, qualified social worker, registered and licensed psychotherapist

This book is an important contribution in the conversation on how mindfulness and compassion can assist people suffering from trauma. It helps to bridge the divide between those of us who are involved with contemplative practises for healing and those of us who need assistance in working through trauma. Well worth making the effort of reading, contemplating and applying.

Barbara Jones, retired lawyer with 40 years of meditation experience

The whole book illustrates the compassion and carefulness that are emphasised as key aspects of the encounter with traumatised people. The theory sections are written on the basis of wide-ranging knowledge, and framed by extensive clinical experience. The tone of these sections encourages you to keep reading, although the content of the book is intermittently unbearable. By the time you get to the last page, you have learnt a great deal.

Lena Malmberg, licensed and registered psychologist and psychotherapist, specialist in clinical psychology

'Understanding complex traumatisation and dissociation is not easy. This book is based on various authentic stories, which are well substantiated with facts about trauma and dissociation, and with accounts of treatment and current research. Thus, it can provide concrete support for those who meet traumatised people in their work.'

Fredrik Garpe, licensed and registered psychologist, licensed and registered psychotherapist and specialist in trauma and dissociation

LIVE NOW

ON TRAUMA AND DISSOCIATION

CHRISTINA LEJONÖGA

ANNICA LILJA LJUNG

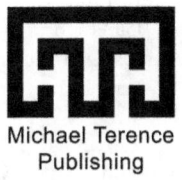

Michael Terence
Publishing

First published in English by
Michael Terence Publishing in 2019
www.mtp.agency

First published in Swedish in 2018 as
Leva Nu - om trauma & dissociation

Authorized translation

Copyright © 2019 Christina Lejonöga and Annica Lilja Ljung

Christina Lejonöga and Annica Lilja Ljung
have asserted the right to be identified as the
authors of this work in accordance with the
Copyright, Designs and Patents Act 1988

ISBN 9781913289683

All rights reserved. No part of this publication may be reproduced,
stored in a retrieval system, or transmitted,
in any form or by any means, electronic, mechanical,
photocopying, recording or otherwise,
without the prior permission of the publisher

Cover image from a painting by Gabriella Luttrup

Interior images by
Elina Ehn
Annica Lilja Ljung
Arne Ljung

Cover design by Michael Terence Publishing

With compassion to you who struggle to overcome trauma and all who care about you…

CONTENTS

FOREWORD 1

AUTHORS' PREFACE 3

CHAPTER 1 5
   Trauma and dissociation meet compassion 5
      Six living stories 5
      Compassion and hope 6
      About the authors 7
      Integration and dissociation 8
      How does dissociation work? 8
      PTSD and DID 9
      From one person to another 9
      Into the light 10
      Who was this book written for? 10

CHAPTER 2 12
   Welcome to our world 12

CHAPTER 3 14
   Putting ourselves in their place 14
      'It can't be true' 14

CHAPTER 4 16
   Our capacity for compassion: an asset 16
      Reading with compassion 16
      Verbal limitations 17
      When we think we know what it's like 17
      Training compassion, awareness and not judging 18
      Being here, wherever you go 19

CHAPTER 5 21
   A simple theoretical basis: trauma and dissociation 21
      Wounds 21

>   Hidden trauma..22
>   Islands in the sea..23
>   Not our own fault..23
>   A fragmented personality...24
>   Immense scope for change..25

CHAPTER 6 27

> *Trauma in modern history*... *27*
>   The horrors of war 28
>   PTSD after hidden trauma 28
>   Cast back in time..29
>   Growing knowledge 29
>   Where we are now 30
>   Mistrust persisting today...30

FIRST STORY 32

> *Emma*.. *34*

CHAPTER 7 62

> *Attachment system: the necessary bonds*............................. *62*
>   Will to live..62
>   Lightning reactions 63
>   Importance of security...63
>   Patterns can change 64
>   Four attachment patterns 65
>   Insecure attachment 66
>   Chaotic attachment..66
>   The infant's inner world..67
>   Imprinted patterns...68
>   Drops eroding stone...69

SECOND STORY 70

> *Christine*... *72*

CHAPTER 8 81

> *Threat system and other action systems*................................ *81*
>   Flee, fight or play dead..81
>   Our inner systems..82
>   Trauma-generated imbalance 82

CHAPTER 9 83

Post-traumatic stress *83*
    Secure enough to cope 83
    We react differently 84
    It happened to me 85
    The PTSD diagnosis 85
    Many different symptoms 86
    Triggers 86
    Insecurity's icy grip 87

THIRD STORY 88
    Oscar *90*

CHAPTER 10 109
Degrees of traumatisation *109*
    Three phases 110
    Traumatisation hard to measure 111
    Trauma-related dissociative disorder 112
    Red alert 112
    Shrinking hippocampus 113
    Fragmented inner world 114
    No interconnection 115
    Ego states and parts of the personality 116
    Locked in a dark wardrobe 117

FOURTH STORY 118
    Yasmine *120*

CHAPTER 11 139
A function for every dissociative part *139*
    Everyday part of the personality — ANP 139
    Survival part of the personality — EP 140
    Examples of survival parts of the personality 140
    Several everyday parts of the personality 141
    Splitting varies in depth 141
    Flashbacks 142
    As if the danger were present now 143
    Everyday life 143
    The most severe results 144
    Second chance in life 145
    Confused terms: schizophrenia, MPD and DID 145
    Psychotic or not? 146

CHAPTER 12 148

Using compassion, self-compassion and mindfulness................................ 148
   The crucial meeting 148
   Aware with the senses 149
   Identifying the problems 150
   The path to successful treatment 150
   'It happened to me, but that was then' 151

FIFTH STORY 152

Joanna 154

CHAPTER 13 189

The whole person needs help 189
   Dissociation: simultaneously knowing and not knowing 189
   Everyone must join in 190
   Warning 190
   Arduous process 191
   Every symptom needs treating 192
   Key crossroads for therapists 192
   Compassion 193
   Building bridges 194
   Destructive acts 194
   Responding to the victim role 195
   Step by step 196
   Phases of trauma therapy 196
   The parts' tug-of-war 197
   Balancing act 198
   Overcoming resistance 199
   Inner minefield 199
   What the hell happened? 200
   Meeting of parts 201
   Wordless speech 201
   Focusing on the body 202
   Can anyone love me? 203
   Mind, consciousness and its nature 204
   Trained awareness: a key to health 205
   East meets West 205
   Awareness 207
   Honest with oneself 207
   Training compassion 208

SIXTH STORY 210
Felicity *212*

CHAPTER 14 252
Ground-breaking research on repercussions of trauma *252*
DID: more common than we think 252
Eminent trauma researcher..252
Research findings: essential reading for doubters 254
The next phase...255
PTSD and DID — deviations on the same scale 256
More than our brain cells 257
Brain activity and reaction time.......................................258
Neutral face frightening 259
Important feelings...260
From science to therapy...260
Memories fall into place 261

CHAPTER 15 262
Last but not least: the costs of treatment...............................*262*
Costs and benefits 263
Correct treatment saves suffering and money 263
Case 1: Lottie — 11 years on the healthcare merry-go-round 263
Case 2: Mary — pain, eating disorders, suicide attempts.............264
Case 3: Louise — the right help early on 265
Financial comparison: major differences..............................265
Diagnosis, treatment and costs 265
Quality of life 266
Everyone gains from the right treatment 266
Hope bounces back 266

LAST WORDS... 270

WHOLEHEARTED THANKS 274

GLOSSARY 277

TRAUMA SCALE 292

GROUP MANUALS 293

WANT TO READ MORE? 294

FOREWORD

Ellert R. S. Nijenhuis is a Dutch psychologist, psychotherapist and researcher. For more than 30 years, he has diagnosed and treated patients suffering from complex traumatisation. He is also a teacher and author of extensive works about trauma-related dissociation and dissociative syndromes.

This book adds to emergent literature showing that, with adequate therapy, even chronically and severely traumatised individuals can heal their wounds. Effective treatment nonetheless demands awareness that the damage incurred by them is more complex than in post-traumatic stress disorder (PTSD) as such. Moreover, it calls for a sensitive, egalitarian and gradual approach where the patient and clinician are equal partners rather than follower and leader respectively.

In part, the complexity of chronically traumatised individuals stems from attachment and separation phobias combined. Children have an unconditional evolutionary need for attachment to their parents and other significant adults. A child's yearning and quest for attachment clashes head-on with fear of these far more powerful people in the event of physical and emotional maltreatment, sexual abuse and emotional neglect. The outcome is a huge conflict that a chronically traumatised child can hardly resolve: between an aching need for the adult to stay and a wish, out of sheer terror, to be left alone. More often than not, this conflict persists into adulthood, making a therapeutic relationship characterised by trust and collaboration elusive.

When survivors understand and overcome prolonged childhood abuse, cruelty and neglect, the benefits reach far beyond them personally. Traumatisation, a massive social and societal problem, challenges family members, professionals and the community at large. Our challenge is to grasp, prevent and remedy its short- and long-term impact on mental and physical health.

This book provides chronically traumatised individuals' personal accounts of the horrors they have endured, and in particular their paths to healing. The moving narratives alternate with lucid theoretical reasoning and down-to-earth descriptions of trauma survivors' mental and physical experiences, symptoms, disturbances and treatment. Compassion and warmth permeate the book.

Together, the authors have created a clear, ethical text that will enrich and inspire a wide audience. I therefore wholeheartedly recommend this remarkable collaborative work to traumatised people and their families, psychologists, psychiatrists, psychotherapists, social workers, doctors, physiotherapists, lawyers, police officers and all others who come into contact with, and care about, individuals who have long been uncherished. My hope is that the book, in view of its importance, will be translated into the world's major languages. The topic deserves no less.

Ellert R. S. Nijenhuis, PhD
November 2019

AUTHORS' PREFACE

Is it possible to heal deep traumas?

How can society provide better support for people who have survived traumas?

And how can we help, so that those who are traumatised are no longer neglected and silenced?

What role do compassion and self-compassion play in their prospects of recovery?

Can work to help enhance their awareness, orientation in time and connection between mind and body promote healing from trauma?

Our aim with the book *Live Now: On Trauma and Dissociation* is to uncover the experience of traumatised fellow human beings and spread awareness of the far-reaching consequences of trauma. The book's six main narrators share their long, arduous struggle to break the shackles of trauma and, step by step, achieve a healthy life. Graphically, exposing the pain, each story is told. These potent testimonies give us a deeper understanding of what a life shaped by powerlessness, abuse, violence or other gruelling experiences may mean.

As the stories illustrate, traumatisation can be exceedingly multifaceted. There is nothing sensational in writing about what it entails: severe suffering, the intrinsic strategies we humans may adopt when we are subjected to trauma, or the long, laborious road to healing. Only when we who are around the victims of trauma truly listen, not fending off what happened but allowing ourselves to understand, can we respectfully get on with arranging for them to get help that works. Only then will our society be one that stands up for the equal worth of every human being.

Each treating psychotherapist needs to have one foot in the traumatised person's world, with deep compassion, and the other standing firmly on well-founded theory. Then we see what we can do to help. The survivors get an honest chance to free themselves from their painful experiences and start living a balanced life.

Sadly, traumatisation is a huge and neglected social problem. Traumatised people are a highly disadvantaged group. There are few treatment options, although the biopsychosocial theory underpinning this book provides sound guidelines. Many sufferers are alone, misinterpreted and deprived of assistance. Our deepest wish is to raise the voices of the traumatised and improve their chances of invariably meeting with respect and compassion, whether they have wounds that can heal relatively fast or that have already developed into major, multilayered trauma.

You, the book's main narrators, show that even deep wounds can heal when trauma survivors are given the right help. We thank you for sharing so bravely, and for spreading hope.

This book was published in Sweden in 2018. The first edition sold out quickly and the book has been reprinted in Swedish. We are very happy that our book will now reach English-speaking readers throughout the world. Trauma exists in every country and the need for healing is worldwide.

We are pleased to see how well this book has been received by its readers in Sweden. This applies to trauma survivors as well as professionals. Many have contacted us. Thank you for valuable feedback and positive contacts. It gives us great joy that our written words come in handy.

Warm thanks for reading our book. Together we create change.

Christina Lejonöga and Annica Lilja Ljung
November 2019

CHAPTER 1

Trauma and dissociation meet compassion

Being human can be wonderful. It can also be very, very difficult. How painful it can be comes across in this book, but its pages are also filled with hope.

An insecure childhood characterised by violence and abuse leaves deep wounds. Traumatic memories do not fade away. They live on in us, in our bodies, affecting our lives.

Six living stories

We can never relive our childhood, nor our teenage years. What we can do as adults, on the other hand, is to build up the security and identity we never had the chance to develop while we were growing up. This makes it possible for even our very deepest wounds to heal.

The people you will meet in this book have achieved it. They were all traumatised when they sought treatment. Each and every one was struggling to overcome personal circumstances and a constantly active past. For some of them, life was an inferno, full of pain, chaos and terror.

Now, with courage and strength, they want to share their life stories. They tell them in the hope that other victims will find the fortitude, energy and willpower to tackle the arduous task of freeing themselves from their own past, so that they can live a healthy life.

This is undeniably a book that describes pain, but it says at least as much about inner human strength. The narrators' own stories have pride of place. Through interviews, six trauma survivors get their own voice. These are potent stories, some characterised by brutality, anguish and suicide attempts, but also by turning points. Since then, they have succeeded in making a good life for themselves.

Today, they all live harmonious lives. They are friendly, warm, thoughtful and compassionate towards themselves and others. Most have fully achieved, and one is very close to, a sound and salubrious existence. Their stories show that even very severely traumatised people can free themselves from their painful past and create a richly rewarding life, here and now. All six express a strong wish to inspire others in trauma, past or present, with hope that they too can achieve joy in life.

Compassion and hope

Severely traumatised people are often extremely quick to blame themselves. The inner critic is sternly judgemental, and self-esteem very weak. The rapid onslaught of harsh, rejecting, often scornful and constantly critical thoughts exerts destructive control over almost every chance of a positive experience or encounter with others. The ability to feel compassion for oneself is often completely non-existent. However, we can all develop our capacity for compassion and self-compassion. Cramping convictions, such as *I am helpless and weak*, can successively give way to strengthening self-images like *I am strong and can take care of myself*.

The therapy received by the people in this book is based on the healing power of compassion. Every moment filled with compassion affects the person who experiences it. Training one's ability to feel compassion towards oneself and others plays a crucial role in healing. Such a process is, of course, characterised by an uncertain dance between trust and insecurity: how can you trust anyone when you have been so mistreated? Nonetheless, the patients have gradually ventured to go all the way, trust the trauma therapist and bond in an atmosphere of compassion. At the same time, this book's narrators have also gradually, step by step, learnt to feel compassion towards themselves. In several of the stories, they relate that compassion and self-compassion were feelings they did not truly know could exist, either in themselves or between people.

Compassion is a recurrent theme throughout the book, and a precondition for hope. Where there is compassion, hope often arises. The sense that *I'm damaged forever* is replaced by the considerably more buoyant feeling of *I'm fine and can get well*. Later on, there is more to tell about this conscious foundation, what compassion actually means and how to practise compassion and self-compassion.

About the authors

Books in this field tend to be either biographies or non-fiction. Here, we link people's unique personal stories with theory, facts and research. We, the authors of this book, are Christina Lejonöga, a journalist, and Annica Lilja Ljung, a licensed and registered therapist. Each of us has personally experienced several traumatic events.

Christina sees her writing as social work in the form of social criticism, in which she highlights victims who otherwise inhabit the shadows. She attaches great importance to recording their messages in a manner as close to their own truth as could ever be achieved. During a long series of interviews, Christina has listened to the stories of the stricken and chosen to express them in the first person, to truly give voice to their experiences. All the interviewees have read their own narratives and confirmed that these, in their view, are correct.

They have all had psychotherapy with Annica, who has worked with traumatised people in various ways for nearly all her working life. A licensed and registered therapist with a degree in social work, she specialises in trauma and dissociation. She is passionate about the subject and helping those who are affected. Now, she wants to share valuable knowledge, both her own and, above all, that of her expert teachers and colleagues, and recent ground-breaking research. For many years she has practised yoga and meditation, which involves exploring various states of consciousness and provides ample training in deep compassion. She finds this practice highly beneficial in her work with traumatised people, and she sees compassion, self-compassion, awareness and body-mind integration as an important foundation for healing and health.

In the stories below, Annica is referred to as 'TT' (short for 'trauma therapist'). We wish to underline that our choice to interview people who have had therapy specifically with Annica was for reasons of trust. They might just as well have been treated by another competent therapist specialising in trauma and dissociation. In the personal stories, the designation 'TT' thus stands for Annica, since it is the narrators' meeting with her, in particular, that they are describing. Our aim is to emphasise that all the narrators' personal development sprang entirely from their own potential.

Integration and dissociation

Before you read on, we want to give you a brief introduction to dissociation.

Every one of us is born with a natural urge to integrate our experiences into a coherent perception of who we are. Our sense of self evolves step by step: *All my thoughts, feelings, sensations and memories belong to me, however wonderful or terrible they are. I am me.*

The opposite of this integration is dissociation. Childhood trauma can deeply damage our ability to perceive ourselves as unified individuals in our own right. Without integration, dissociative parts of the personality can form.

How does dissociation work?

When you have no means of avoiding danger, you adapt and protect yourself as best you can. This can be expressed in 'hiding' mentally — fleeing from your emotions when staying in them feels too overwhelmingly unpleasant. This may be acute or chronic. Dissociation in trauma involves inadequate personality integration. You become detached from the here and now, but when the dissociation comes from trauma it includes disconnection within the whole person. This prevents the trauma from flooding the whole of your consciousness.

Dissociation is like an internal emergency brake that we unconsciously apply to escape from something that is overpowering us. It is an ability we all have and use, but that develops further, and with great ingenuity, if we grow up in a dangerous environment. Dissociation emerges so that we can escape being present in our own body while the horrific event is happening. In its most severe form, dissociation leads to the disintegration of the personality into two or more dissociative parts that coexist within one and the same person.

The process is incessant, even when the danger is over. If you are a survivor you may, in adulthood, get far away from the perpetrator(s) and in fact be safe, but you do not grasp the fact. On the contrary, you keep trying to stay in control of everything around you, with the same intensity and in the same way as when the violence and abuse were being committed. This is not because you choose to do so, but because you have had no help in understanding, on every level, that the danger is actually past. Everything that is happening in the present merges, in a mighty mix-up with what happened before. Chaos rules in your perceptions.

PTSD and DID

'Dissociation' may refer to a single symptom, but can also manifest itself in multiple ways. This is what happens in trauma-related dissociation, and is what this book is about. The dissociation then becomes more pervasive throughout the person, and is termed a syndrome. The severest form is known as Dissociative Identity Disorder (DID).

The people you will meet in this book represent various degrees of traumatisation, from post-traumatic stress disorder (PTSD) to grave forms of dissociation. All of them have struggled for release from the prison of traumatisation. Early in life, many of them have experienced extreme terror, powerlessness and threats to their lives.

To survive, they have developed several more or less isolated portions of their personality, like small islands in an ocean. Various dissociative parts of the personality can take command of a person's behaviour, perceptions and emotions. Memories devoid of context live on as if they are still happening. Further on in this book, you can read more about various degrees of dissociation.

There is nothing spectacular about this human survival mechanism. We might be described as ingeniously designed. Dissociation truly serves its purpose, as long as the danger persists. After that, the victim needs other people's help to realise that the danger is no longer there.

From one person to another

The stories are mainly written in the present tense. Names of people, places and the like have been changed to allow the interviewees to remain anonymous. Since the stories are based on interviews conducted towards the end of the treatment, once integration was complete, fully exposing how the person's chaotic, split inner world was like before and during treatment has not been feasible.

Each person's story is told without comments. This is because the last thing we want is for the readers to pigeonhole the narrators. Instead, we would like them to meet the narrators and their stories as open, compassionate fellow humans.

Some of the terms and concepts in this book may be new to you. A glossary, containing brief explanations, is provided at the end.

Into the light

Our primary purpose in *Live Now: On Trauma and Dissociation* is to provide space for the interviewees' life stories, told by them personally. In so doing, we seek to highlight their fortitude and hard work and to show humankind's astonishing healing capacity. Our secondary purpose is to demonstrate what enormous transformational forces are contained in true compassion and self-compassion.

Severely traumatised people often possess an unused ability to recover. This vulnerable group should be given more scope and the right resources in the community, in the care sector and in their daily lives.

People's behaviour and feelings that stem from trauma must not be reduced to black-and-white discussions of what is true or false. Legal processes can never produce proof that profound, complex psychological conditions do not exist. Nor, obviously, should poorly managed, substandard legal investigations and processes be confused with qualitatively good psychotherapeutic processes.

Our motive for writing this book is to raise the voices of the traumatised and improve their prospects of being treated with respect and compassion. We must not allow people with trauma to be silenced, as they have been so much throughout history and are still being to this day. All these hours' work, the interviewing and writing, are worthwhile if the result is a single other severely traumatised person who gets the right treatment, is helped out of the mental prison of traumatisation and can finally experience the healing power of compassion.

Who was this book written for?

Everyone interested.

Perhaps you too, like the people in this book, have been traumatised, or know someone who has had similar experiences or who you think behaves unusually and has undergone terrible experiences. It might be someone in your family, your girlfriend or boyfriend, a close friend, colleague, childhood friend...

Perhaps you are reading the book because you meet people with mental problems in your work. You may be a psychotherapist, psychologist, doctor, nurse, midwife, social worker, therapy assistant, priest or teacher. Whether you work at a health centre, in occupational healthcare, at a social security office or job centre or elsewhere, and if you come into contact with many people, we believe you will benefit from our book. Wherever you are, you may encounter men and women who are shaped by traumatic experiences and sometimes react in apparently odd ways.

CHAPTER 2

Welcome to our world

Six people; six life stories. These are the interviewees you will meet in this book.

Emma

Emma grows up with a deeply depressed mother and a father who imposes harsh rules. Emma longs to be loved, but her parents neglect her and she feels invisible.

'Walking by the water is just for happy people. I'm not worth going there. That's how I used to feel. Today, I know I've got a right to be alive.'

Christine

Christine loses her son in an accident. The shock causes her to shut down her feelings. Instead of mourning and moving on in life, her heart remains mute.

'Suddenly death snatches away my beloved child. The whole future with him just disappears. I'm shut inside a bubble of locked feelings.'

Oscar

Oscar grows up in what looks like an ordinary family. But under the surface, something is horribly wrong. To survive, he locks up the scared little guy and the angry, powerful boy.

'Dad orders me to lick Mum's genitals. He watches and masturbates. I'm seven or eight years old. Everything's incomprehensible. Part of me dies. It's like living in two different realities. In the daytime, it's ordinary life. In the evening and at night, there are no limits.'

Yasmine

Sexual abuse, inadequate care, betrayal by adults and grief for siblings who took their own lives cause Yasmine's personality to split into several dissociative parts. She ends up in a mental hospital, is pumped full of tablets and gets 52 electrical treatments. No one listens to her.

'I've lost a lot: my childhood, my siblings, my life. Now, at last, I've woken up and don't feel disgusting any more.'

Joanna

Joanna's father abuses her sexually. The incomprehensible acts take place again and again. He takes his daughter to other adults who violate her. Repeatedly, she is severely assaulted and beaten.

'I can't escape. To protect myself, I flee from reality. It's like disappearing into a black hole. Separate parts of me have to bear the pain and terror. I live in an inner chaos with 16 different parts of my personality, all pulling in their own directions.'

Felicity

Felicity's father shot and killed her mother, and was sent to a high-security psychiatric unit. After two years in family care homes, the children were taken from the safety of their foster parents' care and placed with their father.

'I'm forced to live with my mom's killer. It's a grim upbringing that drives me straight into the arms of a deadly dangerous man. Reality's unbearable. No wonder I disappear into myself.'

CHAPTER 3

Putting ourselves in their place

Now you have glimpsed the people you will meet in this book. We ask you to read their life stories with empathy, sympathy and, above all, real compassion. Let yourself linger in the encounter with each narrator. Allowing ourselves to be deeply moved, we can grasp the gigantic scale of the task and what admirable progress these people are making, despite the echoing pain of their past.

We all have a desire to be happy, share in what is good and simply enjoy life. Usually, we want to avoid all emotional experiences that are negative. We automatically try to rid ourselves of painful feelings, and have no wish to feel shame, grief, anger, aversion, frustration, jealousy, envy or discontent. Nor do we want to feel sad and gloomy. Nonetheless, we do — all of us. Bearing such feelings calls for immense effort. That is why it is easy for us to stop reading when something feels unpleasant. But we ask you, who are now holding this book in your hand, to find out what stories these people have to tell. They are worth it.

'It can't be true'

Try to read with awareness, let yourself be emotionally involved, and stay with your reactions despite the unpleasant feelings they cause. Our wish is for you to connect the factual knowledge with emotional understanding. The text requires it.

There is always a risk of us rejecting the painful side of life — being unable or unwilling to take it in. Usually, we intellectualise or distance ourselves, thereby protecting ourselves from people's harsh life stories. We then join in creating the fate that afflicts traumatised people worldwide. We fend off the pain, question it and sometimes even deny its credibility or truth. If, instead, we read with fortitude and compassion, it helps these individuals and all the other traumatised people in the world.

When you let compassion fill you entirely with a genuine desire to ease the suffering of others, compassion spreads around you in all directions.

The book shows that hard work makes it possible to move on in life, despite devastatingly painful experiences and perhaps a very poor start. It shows that leading a happy and healthy life and overcoming severe trauma are feasible. If you are yourself traumatised in a similar way to the narrators, read the book in smaller portions. Create some distance, so that you do not become overwhelmed. And if you are not already getting it, seek professional help.

CHAPTER 4

Our capacity for compassion: an asset

The book's main narrators relate their thoughts, feelings and memories, along with an account of their personal development and life situation. Their candid stories remind us how vulnerable we humans are. We hope that they set off an echo within you that is allowed to reverberate, deepening your understanding of what life is and has been like for many people.

The stories show that, by making efforts, we humans are fully capable of achieving the security and identity we never had the chance to develop while growing up. With the right support as adults, we can create the necessary building blocks that may be missing from our childhood. Then we can heal even the deepest of wounds.

Reading with compassion

The people you meet in the book were suffering from varying degrees of severity on the 'trauma scale', and met the criteria for various diagnoses, when they came to the therapist. They had great inner potential, but needed skilled support to find the path to healing through compassion and self-compassion. They all toiled hard, using their abilities and the strength that can grow if other people help. Again and again, and in an admirable way, they have renewed their efforts to take yet another step forward, and eventually overcome their trauma.

Today, they all live harmonious lives. Bravely, they now choose to tell their stories, hoping that other victims will be strong enough to embark on their own demanding journey. And then, when they have freed themselves from the grip of their own personal history, they will at last be able to start living a healthy life.

Verbal limitations

Every chapter you find before, between and after the life stories is independent of the personal testimonies. When the text is at a general and theoretical level, too, we ask you to take time to sometimes pause and try to engage with the stories again, and with your inner reactions.

We humans are very much in the habit of embarking on superficial ways of thinking, sorting concepts into categories and thinking *now we've grasped this, now we know*. But what does this actually mean? What would it have been like for me, if I had been the victim? Perhaps we humans are more equal than we imagine. Perhaps the distance between what we call 'you' and 'me' is shorter than we think. Is this something worth bearing in mind when we create theories and divide ourselves and others into groups? Occasionally, we should ask ourselves: *How do we remain humble, respectful and compassionate when we use theories about what we think others are suffering from?*

When we think we know what it's like

We need to be aware of the sometimes black-and-white theoretical statements that often simplify and impose restrictions. Otherwise, we fall into a trap. *We think we know what something is like because we have labelled it.* We automatically label parts of reality as relating to *'the other person, not me'*, and easily lose true compassion. Our thinking becomes polarised: about 'us' and 'them'.

In medical records, the anamnesis (the patient's history) and diagnoses, such as that of PTSD, are listed. Each is followed by a full stop. Often, there is no reference to what caused the person's symptoms. It might say: 'The patient was subjected to abuse by X during childhood'; but such traumatic events are never mentioned again. Consequences of violence and abuse are disregarded. Of course, traumatisation is not universally dealt with so dismissively in psychiatric records, but this inadequacy is, unfortunately, all too common.

As we noted in the book's introductory chapter, it is the wound that is the trauma, not the actual event(s). The consequences of experiencing abuse and other events must be emphasised. It is the harm, specifically, we need to deal with. Too rarely do people ask themselves: *In what way do the injuries or wounds affect the patient's life? What results do they have today? How do they shape the victim's everyday existence?*

Psychiatric records may contain hundreds of pages about how the patients have behaved, and what symptoms (such as anxiety and depression) they have had, over years of contact. The drugs they have been given to cure or relieve the symptoms are listed. Sometimes, medicines are undoubtedly necessary. It is not a simple truth that a psychotherapeutic treatment alone can solve everything. But do we health professionals perhaps lose the opportunity to provide optimal help if we become too black and white in our way of seeing, objectifying patients from the outside? Maybe we even put ourselves slightly above our patients — our fellow human beings. Perhaps, as professionals, we must have only one foot in theory and let the other take a step into the patient's subjective world to be able to help in providing any real relief and remedy. It may be that we who work with traumatised people must dare to penetrate deep inside ourselves to maintain this balance in a humble way.

Language is a gift and an asset, but simultaneously imposes limitations. We must relate to this when the theories are about people. The Persian poet Rumi expressed it as follows:

'Not the ones speaking the same language, but the ones sharing the same feeling, understand each other.'

Training compassion, awareness and not judging

We shall begin by describing why compassion, self-compassion, mindfulness and integration of body and mind can be a good basis for treating traumatised people. As we have noted, severely traumatised people are quick to judge themselves, and they may entirely lack the ability to feel inwardly directed compassion. With multiple dissociative parts of the personality inside, there are additional major difficulties.

The positive aspect is that we can all develop our capacity for compassion and self-compassion. Developing this ability plays a key role in the treatment. The therapist helps patients to understand themselves and the dissociative parts of their personalities; to develop a team inside themselves; and to create an inner world based on compassion and respect among the various parts. Being able to let kindness and compassion gradually emerge among the parts needs practice in taking a balanced view, accepting views other than one's own and enduring overwhelming bodily reactions and emotion.

Slowly, we create access to compassion inside the victim. This, we argue, is the most important building block for all human coexistence. Compassion facilitates future integration of the whole personality. Understandably, the victim has become fragmented inside by the friction, and often a complete lack of compassion, among the dissociative parts of the personality.

Being here, wherever you go

One component of the treatment received by the traumatised patients you are meeting in the book has been mindfulness practice. Around the world, research on mindfulness is under way. Brain research in recent years has pointed to a number of its positive effects on the human brain. Practising mindfulness helps to synchronise the brain's various components by, for example, reducing stress, worry and suffering, improving emotional balance and increasing the ability to stay in the body and cope with pain.

For traumatised patients, this practice needs to be undertaken cautiously and gently. It is important for it to include the aspect of not judging oneself. Awareness of one's thoughts and feelings in the present moment, along with the ability to choose an attitude of acceptance towards these thoughts and feelings, can be a great help to people suffering from traumas.

By practising mindfulness, compassion and self-compassion with trauma sensitivity and sometimes individually designed guidance, the patients can boost the recovery of their central nervous system. They gradually become more comprehensible to themselves and can, step by step, put a facilitative distance between themselves and their own thoughts and feelings. This is conscious practice to change accustomed patterns, not essentially to create serenity or to enter into any other states of consciousness — simply to alter the 'well-trodden' paths in the brain and body.

The practice must be undertaken with care. Standardised instructions, such as *Sit on a cushion* and *Follow your breathing*, risk generating more anxiety, racing thoughts or dissociation. To be beneficial, meditation often needs to be adapted to the practitioners individually, in the phase they have reached. The exercises should emphasise different things for different people on different occasions. The scholar and trauma professional David A. Treleaven has studied the knowledge gaps in Vipassanā (the name means 'seeing things as they really are'), the global meditation movement in the Buddhist tradition. These gaps relate to the needs of traumatised people who take part in retreats. His study provides support for meditation practice to be adapted to each person's circumstances and needs. After ten years of research he is offering a program designed to support those who want to be informed about the potential pitfalls of mindfulness meditation for trauma survivors.

Further on in the book, we shall return to the significance of compassion. The next chapter focuses on the notions of trauma and dissociation.

CHAPTER 5

A simple theoretical basis: trauma and dissociation

This chapter explains traumatisation, in particular its severe form, and structural dissociation. Making these highly complex phenomena readily understandable is a challenge. Our ambition is to create a book everyone finds readable, where self-experienced personal stories have pride of place and patients themselves describe the recovery process, but insight into complex theories is also provided.

We start by describing trauma and dissociation. Further on, we look more closely at attachment theory and how the bonds between caregivers and children influence the latter's development and mental health. We choose to write about the attachment system because this action system has such a big impact on our lives.

Wounds

Trauma means 'wound'. Psychological wounds result from events we experience as overwhelming. The trauma is the injury itself, not the actual event(s). We all have minor, everyday wounds that have affected our mindset. These, however, heal. But the traumatising wounds are so deep that, even long afterwards, the bleeding does not stop. They do not heal. The pain continues to torment us.

In many ways, we humans are very much alike. We have the same basic needs: food, sleep, water and warmth in a loving embrace. From birth, we need close attachment to adults who take care of us, see and understand our signals, and give us love and protection. We need security, both external and internal.

The newborn human is one of Earth's most vulnerable young creatures. Home is supposed to be our safe place. Our close relationships need to nurture us, enabling us to grow into secure individuals. Most children who suffer the occasional trauma and receive support and help cope with it very well.

Inadequate security intensifies vulnerability. Recurrent harsh events in childhood exacerbate the traumatisation risk, especially if relationships with our caregivers give us no security. Once again: in secure conditions, traumatic childhood wounds can heal very well. But suffering terror and other frightening emotions repeatedly, *without* being soothed and affirmed, gives us no basis for security. If we have the misfortune of frequently suffering from poor care, emotional coldness, neglect or rejection, if we witness or are subjected to violence or sexual abuse, or if perhaps we are even assaulted by someone close to the defenceless person we are, the risk of complicated forms of traumatisation increases.

Hidden trauma

If the perpetrator is the father, mother or some other adult on whom the child depends, the trauma is doubled. To survive, we are compelled to keep looking to these people. We live in constant, questioning uncertainty. *Will I get beaten or caressed?* The home becomes a minefield. *Where do I dare to tread?*

Moving away from home is not an option. Children stay and try, in every way, to adjust and adapt their conduct according to whatever they can think of doing to avoid attack. They want to hide and forget what they have suffered. The child may be intimidated into silence. The trauma becomes unmentionable: a well-hidden secret. Other people's inability or reluctance to see reality as it is and help the child is devastating. Abandonment and silence further aggravate the risk of grave psychological damage, or what may be called 'biopsychosocial wounds'.

Gradually, the child's abilities grow. The brain and body develop. *Where* in this process the child undergoes traumatising events has a bearing on the aftermath of the trauma. Many survivors of grim circumstances that include constant abuse make use of their own diverse abilities. They develop, for example, good study skills, sensitivity in reading other people's subtle signals, verbal proficiency, tenacity, cunning and many other traits. But when the brain develops under such conditions, the part that evolved to protect us becomes hypersensitive and overly dominant in relation to the brain's other areas.

Islands in the sea

Our experiences shape who we become as people. We are born into differing environments and cannot affect the conditions we grow up in. The long-term stress imposed on us by repeated severe events early in life is easy to understand. That this can even alter brain structure is considerably less known.

Our early relationships affect how our brain develops and our well-being later in life. We are shaped particularly by what happens to us in our first few years, when the brain is most malleable. The stories in this book are evidence of very severe cases of traumatisation. Many of the interviewees were overwhelmed at an early age by gruelling experiences and feelings that they had no means of coping with. Horrific memories, with no context, live on as if they are still happening. To survive, the child may develop several dissociative parts of the personality, like small islands in an ocean. Why does this happen?

Not our own fault

As previously noted, we adapt and protect ourselves as best we can when we have no way of avoiding the danger. Distancing ourselves from the here and now, we flee from the terror and all the overwhelming emotions, disconnecting from reality. We dissociate, going into mental 'hiding' so that the trauma cannot reach throughout our consciousness.

Dissociation may be compared to an emergency brake inside us: unconsciously, we use it to save ourselves from a situation that overpowers us. Dissociation develops because we cannot be present in the body while the overwhelmingly horrific event is taking place. As Judith Lewis Herman (psychiatrist and psychotherapist) expresses it, *'This altered state of consciousness might be regarded as one of nature's small mercies, a protection against unbearable pain.'*

We humans do all we can to cope with life's difficulties: our best, based on our own circumstances. The brain adapts to and is shaped by our strategies. Even when everything around us changes over time, our brain continues to use tried and tested patterns from our earlier life. Strategies that helped us in childhood cause major problems now, in adulthood.

Adult trauma survivors with these problems are encountered by professionals in the care sector. Deep listening makes these victims' 'incomprehensible' behaviours, feelings and thoughts highly understandable. They are neither insane nor unintelligible; and they are fully treatable. We wish to emphasise the tremendous potential often found in traumatised people who get the right help.

A fragmented personality

Thus, within the child, several dissociative parts of the personality may evolve. Overwhelming experiences from the past live on as if they are occurring now. The parts carry different memories, behaviours and feelings: some know what has taken place and still believe that the awfulness is happening now, while others have no contact with the same memory.

If the abuse begins early in life, the newborn infant's fragmented world never gets a chance to merge together as the child grows up. There is no personality integration. Instead, the small islands are manifested, isolated from one another at least to some extent. This fragmentation becomes a way of taking a break from the experience of terrible, traumatising events. If these events are absent from a specific 'island', it may be possible to go to school, rest and engage in daily life with friends. On another 'island', the child sees new attacks looming if an adult's tone of voice or facial expression, for example, triggers an experience of trauma.

The result is deficient, or dissociative, integration of personality. When this happens, the whole person is incapable of correct orientation in time. Present and past are mixed together. In adulthood, too, there are still dissociative parts of the personality that perceive that the previous hazardous existence is still going on, although in reality the person has long since escaped from the danger. These different parts can live in conflict with one another, and often have divergent solutions to how things should be done. Life becomes chaotic.

Immense scope for change

The brain is plastic. Severe trauma early in life can alter the brain's development potential and lead to trauma-related dissociation.

At the same time, the fact that the brain and body change depending on how we use them offers hope. It gives us prospects and opportunities of repairing old injuries and transforming our lives. Despite their painful experiences, traumatised people, too, can be enabled by proper therapeutic treatment to transcend their limitations, leave their history behind and build new inner security.

Below in this book, we describe in more detail what actually happens in the brain and body when trauma results in dissociation and how we humans, thanks to the brain's healing ability, can develop far more than we ever thought possible.

The stories related here are compelling evidence that healing is fully achievable. But it demands a great deal from the care services. To provide correct treatment, it is vital to be able to assess how traumatised a person is. If professionals diagnose post-traumatic stress disorder (simple PTSD), and initiate treatment for this, when the person is actually suffering from a more intractable trauma-related dissociative disorder, healing may fail to occur. At worst, the patient may be harmed.

This book should, we hope, enhance understanding of complex traumatisation and dissociation. As the stories it contains bear witness, prospects of recovery are very good. Our wish is for many more people to want to join good cooperative partnerships with traumatised people on their necessary and arduous journey forward to a viable, happy life.

We would like to emphasise the importance of striving for continuity in contact with trauma patients. It is in secure relationships that survivors have the opportunity to develop and become healthy. Contacts with professionals therefore need to be lasting: otherwise, healing may not happen. At worst, termination of therapeutic contacts triggers bad old memories or patterns. Changes are sometimes required, of course; in life, things happen to professionals too. But we should always strive to truly minimise discontinuity of care contacts.

CHAPTER 6

Trauma in modern history

History features recurrent periods when the existence of psychological trauma is ignored. A quick retrospect of the western world shows that studies relating to psychological trauma have periodically fallen into oblivion. In the 19th century, several people researched trauma, but their results were abruptly discarded. Classic documents have been written, but treated as inconsequential. On and off, some of the theories have been updated.

Without exploring why, we note here that prevailing professional and social interests affect whether mental wounds and their consequences are neglected. Established society then refuses to give credence to the importance of trauma. Patients' testimonies are labelled 'fantasies' or deemed insignificant.

One of Sigmund Freud's early writings from the late 19th century was about people exposed to extreme stress in the form of sexual abuse. The women's mental problems, dubbed 'hysteria', were associated with gross assaults and abuse. When the rest of the world distanced itself from his theory, Freud made a public apology, declaring that it was not trauma after all that had caused the women's suffering. Instead, he was convinced that the patients' stories were more about fantasies than real experiences.

However, history testifies that psychological trauma always resurfaces, revealed in all its truth. Sooner or later, its consequences need to be tackled. At a time when trauma is recognised and acknowledged, we are struck by shocking insights, which are often succeeded by helplessness. What can we do about the extent of vulnerability and the cruel forms of expression human nature can take?

The horrors of war

War and disasters can cause trauma. In the First World War, there was talk of 'shell-shock syndrome'. After the Second, the diagnoses 'war sailor syndrome' and 'KZ syndrome' (where KZ stood for *Konzentrationslager*, concentration camp) came into being to describe the consequences of camp survivors' trauma. But these diagnoses were swiftly forgotten.

In modern times, the Vietnam War was an important milestone in understanding of psychological trauma. Many American soldiers who experienced the horrors of that war suffered from severe stress. The post-traumatic stress disorder (PTSD) diagnosis was conceived. It acknowledged the severe effects of psychological trauma.

At first, the diagnosis was linked solely to war, disasters and other extreme events beyond our normal life experience. But traumatic events also occur where we are expected to be safe: at home and in our own neighbourhood. Abuse in close relationships becomes, as we have previously noted, a double trauma that challenges a secure worldview. Recognition of the PTSD diagnosis as a result of the Vietnam War meant that the realisation of its similarities to, specifically, the consequences of abuse, threats and violence in the home became unavoidable.

PTSD after hidden trauma

At approximately the same time as PTSD became a recognised diagnosis, psychiatrists Judith Lewis Herman and two colleagues at Boston University Medical Center were investigating people diagnosed with emotionally unstable personality disorder and other identity disorders. The researchers found that these individuals had often been subjected to sexual abuse. The findings circulated underground for several years before the bold step of publishing the conclusions was taken. Once the book finally came out, the link to PTSD was clear. No longer could anyone deny that people exposed to violence and sexual abuse show the same symptoms as traumatised war veterans.

Despite Judith Lewis Herman's and her colleagues' research, changing public awareness has taken a long time. Many continued to associate the PTSD diagnosis with war and disasters. Even in the professional community, this misconception and limitation persisted for a very long time. Gradually, people have been given better support for the suffering inflicted by war. On the other hand, it has been difficult for women, men and children to get the impact of violence and abuse in close relationships and families recognised by society. Silence and denial meet many victims when they seek help. This response lies in the perpetrator's interests and becomes part of the actual assault. It worsens the traumatisation.

Cast back in time

The criteria of the PTSD diagnosis have been revised several times. Currently, people must have experienced, witnessed or been confronted by an event representing a threat to life, threat of serious injury or threat to physical integrity. Alternatively, they may have witnessed someone close to them being subjected to such a specific threat. The focus is on the event having caused intense fear, helplessness or terror.

Crucially, the criterion is that the traumatic events generate symptoms that are experienced as disturbing and painful. This is often a matter of intrusive flashbacks that suddenly cast the traumatised person back to the time and reality when the events took place. The terror reaction is dormant in the body, which is on constant alert. A smell, sound or other sensory impression may suffice to set off the alarm with full force. Mental shutdown can be one reaction. But the symptom profile may also be less clear and avoidance or, for example, physical symptoms may predominate.

Growing knowledge

Extensive studies in the US and elsewhere show that more than half the population have experienced at least one life event of the kind that can cause PTSD. A significant proportion of people have experienced more than one such traumatic event. However, this does not mean that they are all stricken with PTSD. As noted earlier, the trauma is the psychological wound, not the actual event. Those who, after the event, get the right response and good, prompt help in dealing with their experiences do not necessarily develop PTSD.

Research is advancing. It has shown that trauma can lead to both hormonal and structural changes in the brain. Knowledge about complex traumatisation has increased. After multiple traumatic events, perhaps over a prolonged period when the victim's freedom is restricted, and when violence and abuse are intentionally perpetrated in close relationships, the clinical picture becomes more serious. The symptoms are then more numerous and severe, and personality is affected. Victims often live with pain and develop dissociation. Body and consciousness are then separated and are no longer in harmony at all. We return to these more complicated forms of traumatisation below.

Where we are now

For a while now, the western world again seems to have been in an era when psychological trauma is heeded to some extent. What will the outcome of this increased attention be this time? Will society take trauma seriously, try to learn even more, conduct research and make progress? Or will psychological trauma be silenced and watered down because many people are beginning to call every crisis a trauma? Will overdiagnosis and ignorance then be taken as evidence that it is not worth devoting resources and attention to the tribulations of the traumatised? Should people in other occupational categories, such as journalists, be able to act as spokespeople for what trauma can or cannot do to people, so that psychotherapists and doctors are 'dismissed' as experts in their own treatment rooms?

All those who were or had been severely traumatised and who read this book before its original release (in Swedish) have found their way very easily. They understand the processes and confirm that those who deny that the consequences of trauma exist, just as the interviewees describe them, have never listened to a victim sufficiently carefully or sensitively enough, or in the right way.

Mistrust persisting today

One of the traumatised people who test-read our book said:

'A journalist wrote that you can't lose your memory and later get it back. What planet does he live on? He probably didn't realise the memory was never really lost and just hasn't been accessible to me all the time. I also listened to an academic who got everything totally jumbled up. Police interrogations, judgements, psychology and media reporting became one big hotchpotch, which he thought was enough proof that it's impossible for people to have more than one person inside them. It's as if one wrongly handled case were an argument for not listening to the rest of us, who truly know and who may not even have been near a court or anything... We've just been trying to survive all the violence and all the disgusting abuse we've been subjected to.

'Have they considered the fact that they're destroying the situation for us when they state things and speak for all of us, as if they've talked to us? I get so... so... sad.'

To gain further understanding of trauma and dissociation, we must look more closely at how the vital bonds between caregivers and children affect every human being's development. There is an innate need for love and emotional closeness in all of us. When we learn more about how our earliest relationships shape us, we can gain a deeper understanding of how violence, abuse and lovelessness affect our personality and mental health. Further on in the book, we return to the phenomenon of dissociation and discuss various degrees of dissociation in depth.

First, however, it is time to meet Emma.

FIRST STORY

A small child is constantly in a cascade of perceptions. If we are in touch with how we sometimes felt in childhood, we surely all recognise situations when we felt disregarded, abandoned, alone and invisible. We thought we were inadequate — not as good as we should be. At times, we felt that what went on among adults was beyond our understanding.

For children *never* to have such feelings is not possible. Nor can adults correctly interpret every perception and feeling in children, or even see all their reactions. A good parent or caregiver may, at best, succeed in noticing about half of a child's reactions. For adults to see and respond to a child's whole emotional experience is neither feasible nor even desirable.

Children must practise coping with feelings and experiences they do not actually want, and learn that they are part of life. But if feelings of being allowed neither to be seen nor to exist come to dominate a child's thought patterns owing to adults' negligence — perhaps because they are so busy trying to cope with their own concerns and lives — the child suffers a deficit, and damage, as a result.

Emma made initial contact with TT by email: *'A friend recommended you. Can you help me think differently?'* A few years later, she told her story as follows.

Christina Lejonöga : Annica Lilja Ljung

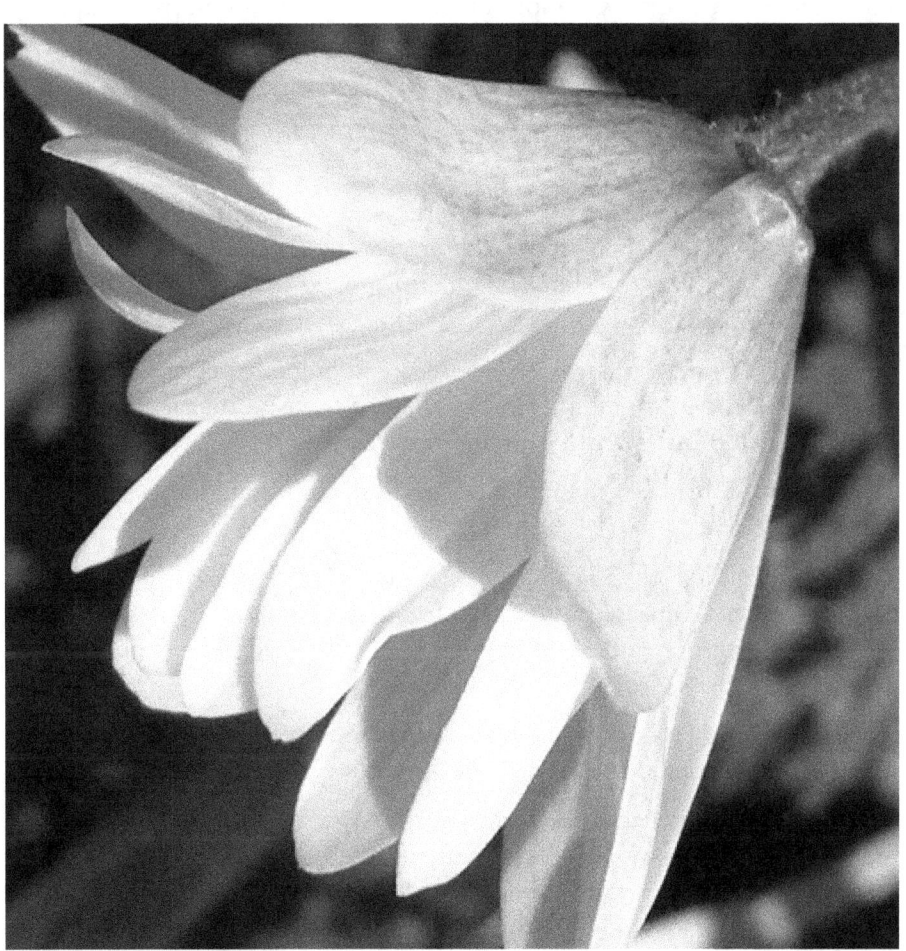

By Elina Ehn, well on the way to health

Emma

I grow up with a deeply depressed mother and a father who imposes extremely harsh rules.

'I long to be loved but feel completely invisible.'

The word 'should' is very important in my life. Throughout my childhood, I was told repeatedly that I should be nice and good — that I shouldn't be a nuisance.

'Svensson's daughters never feel bad. You just need to pull yourself together.' That's what my father said.

I weighed only just over two kilos at birth, and slept a huge lot in my first year of life — an easy baby to look after, who didn't require much attention. So perhaps the shock was all the greater for my parents when I began to explore the world.

They've always said I was wild. Maybe I was trying to catch up on what I'd missed. Dad and Mum didn't want to take me to visit other families. They were ashamed of me — and I took in the shame.

This is how I remember my childhood at home in Aspudden, a Stockholm suburb.

Dad is strict and works a lot; Mum is fragile. Later, I realised she was deeply depressed throughout my childhood. On two occasions, she tried to get treatment but came home again, saying they hadn't been able to help her.

Mum often cries and never takes the initiative. Her crying and Dad's harsh rules leave their mark on me. It's a deep one.

My big sister's four years older than me. We're very different and not close to each other. It always feels like it's my job to make family life run smoothly. It's a heavy responsibility. I try not to disturb anyone — not to be heard, or seen, or to do anything that anyone needs to be ashamed of. I can't remember any feeling of being important in my own right.

Someone else's kid

I'm not scared of people and can talk to anyone. But you're not supposed to do that. If I show anger, I get rejected. I'm invisible. It's just never right for me to come forward. There are no other options. That's just the way it is.

Our parents are self-absorbed to the max. They don't notice me and my feelings. There's no space for my needs. I become good at reading other people, and being obliging.

There's no need for orders. The message comes across anyway, wordlessly: *Don't upset your parents. Do nothing to embarrass them.* When, every so often, I fail to be the invisible child, I'm ashamed. The shame is strong. I feel so bad. I see in their faces, their eyes, that I'm not their child then. I'm just anyone, like someone else's child.

When children in my class are allowed to attend the parents' meeting at school, I have to be 'nice' and sit still with Mum and Dad and all the adults, while my classmates play and are noisy. What I want is never important. All that matters is how Dad wants me to behave, so he doesn't have to be ashamed of me. Running around and having fun with the others just isn't an option.

Dad says: *'I love you as long as you don't do anything you or your parents are ashamed of.'* There's never any unconditional love. I'm afraid of making mistakes and being rejected. I feel vulnerable. How can I know in advance what they might be ashamed of? Best to be invisible...

Dad's girl

When I'm seven, I hear that Dad's sister has 'done herself in'. It was all extremely vague. I don't understand what's happened. In my teens, I hear from a cousin that my aunt has hanged herself in the basement. But that isn't something you can admit. If you're having a hard time, you have to stop thinking about it straightaway. Put a lid on it.

Always trying to be perfect, keep the surface glossy and hide the ugly, disturbing side away takes a lot of effort. But I manage well. I'm well trained. My parents have an easy time with me. Their demands have shaped me like that. I'm simply not allowed to make a fuss.

Dad never raises his voice to me. There's no need. I read the expressions on his face. I see his disgust at other children who behave badly, and I hear him badmouthing them in front of me. 'How can Larry's mother let him run around like that? That really isn't acceptable. Ugh!'

One thing Dad says to me sticks in my heart like a thorn. 'If you'd been our first child, there would never have been any more children. We couldn't take you anywhere because you were so wild.' I swallow his words, deep inside me. I feel ashamed, loathsome and unwanted. I'm Dad's girl and have to behave, so as to be good enough.

To make them like me, I adapt to their expectations. Behave in ways that are rewarded. Avoid doing the kind of thing that's punished with disapproval. Still, I don't feel secure. I feel no warmth, no tenderness.

There's always a distance. I can never sit on their laps. I long constantly for affection, and hope for it intensely. Might I get a hug? Will he put his arms round me, maybe? But no: there are meals on the table and clean clothes for me, but there's no closeness.

Nice and good

I'm left alone with my feelings. Being sad, afraid or angry isn't allowed. It's all ignored. With no affirmation from Mum and Dad, I never learn to understand what I feel. I just get overwhelmed by a jumble of perceptions inside me. It's horrible, so I switch off, stop feeling and become empty.

Dad makes himself extremely clear. He says his daughters and the guys they choose to live with mustn't smoke, drink alcohol, listen to hard rock or dress 'immorally'. Dad's values are explicit and he demands obedience. I never rebel, of course. I don't dye my hair purple or come home with a punk mohawk.

At school I'm a nice, good girl. The teachers see me as a role model and let me take care of new pupils. It becomes my task to keep the class in order. That gives me a certain status, of course, but the coolness factor is low. I'm constantly on my guard with others. I don't strive to join in. Not once does Mum or Dad encourage me to bring a friend home. I just go with the flow.

Darn it, I'm so good at looking happy! Keeping up the façade. Nobody knows how I feel inside. That isn't important.

My big sister Eva's Mum's girl. I'm always Dad's girl. The two of us are totally different — night and day. The fears and everything Dad says flow off Eva like water off a duck's back. In me they go deep and hurt.

There's an empty space between Mum and me. I have no memories of feeling loved. So it feels more important to be liked by Dad. I kind of put him on a pedestal and look up to him. What Dad thinks is what matters most. If I'm quiet and nice he likes me — and I long for that.

Growing silence

My maternal aunt lives in the United States. I like her a lot and come to life when she visits. We meet at Gran and Grandpa's. My aunt, a primary school teacher, gives me scraps of paper she's drawn things on, and then I have to write down what they are called in English. It's great fun.

I enjoy the attention. But Dad puts a stop to it, saying I should understand that I mustn't disturb people. My aunt's on holiday and certainly has more than enough of teaching children in school, he says. That makes me terribly ashamed. I realise that if I assert myself it will cause trouble for someone else.

A couple of years later, my shoulder gets dislocated. Dad takes me to the hospital. When the shoulder has to be twisted back into place, it hurts so much that I give a high-pitched scream. Dad gets angry and tells me to control myself and shut up. I mustn't make trouble for the hospital staff, he says. All he thinks about is what it's like for them, not for me. He doesn't see how terrified I am. I feel abandoned and totally worthless.

Mum is a housewife until my 13th birthday. Our parents live together but still, I can't remember the family ever having a good time together. We never go on an outing to Hellasgården, the forest recreation area, to grill sausages or make shelters. I always played out in the yard.

Mum's at home the whole summer. Why don't we do anything together? It's a mystery. I long so much for us to think of something fun to do, but my attempts to get attention just annoy her.

When I say I'd like to do some baking with Mum, she shows no pleasure; instead, she shows clearly that to her it's just a bore. She's always busy doing what she has to do. Having dinner ready on the table when Dad came home. Cleaning. In my whole childhood, I never saw a single ball of fluff.

We have a caravan, but use it only in the few weeks when Dad's on holiday. We never, ever leave the campsite together to go on a little outing. Mum's always sad and passive. She says it's Dad's fault we never do anything. Even when we go somewhere new, the pattern is exactly the same. Do Mum and Dad like being with us at the campsite? I don't think so…

Green man

Aged 10, I already know our parents will divorce. They say nothing, but I understand anyway. Dad gets his own flat and sometimes retreats there when life gets on top of him. I try even harder to be perfect and fend off the sense of shame.

I'm a weekend child. Although my parents wait till I am 16 to get divorced, I know the relationship is over long before that. They just stick together for the children's sake, as people say.

I often go around with my stomach in knots. When we sit down for dinner, I know in advance it may end with a fight. Although I don't want to hear them quarrelling, I just sit there. Only when I get a bit older do I dare get up and leave the table to avoid witnessing their arguments.

Mum has always been jealous of me because I'm Dad's girl. She tries to start conflicts and provoke Dad. If he says the food's good, she immediately counters with a sour comment: 'Not as good as your mother's cooking, huh?' And then the quarrel gets going.

She clearly shows her displeasure about Dad and me being close. I wish Mum had female friends she could have got support from. But she's lonely and has never had any friends. Instead, she drags us children into the quarrel. I wish Mum hadn't involved me.

As Dad's girl, I'm allowed to go with him to commercial vehicle trade fairs, to admire engines, tractors and so on. Both there and in the city, the message is drummed into me: 'You mustn't get in the drivers' way.'

When I want to cross the street, I definitely mustn't press the button for the green man at the pedestrian crossing, Dad says. It would just make trouble and make it difficult for the drivers. I absolutely mustn't expect them to wait for me. If I ever press the button anyway, I get a strong sense of guilt straightaway, and my self-image becomes ever more negative and destructive.

So embarrassing

Dad gets angry almost every day. Explodes. Shouts 'Bloody hell!' Not at me, but at others, such as other drivers on the road. He's like a powder keg of suppressed anger. He keeps a lid on it until, in the end, there's too much pressure and it goes off with a bang. I find going by car with Dad disagreeable. If anyone hears him, it feels terribly embarrassing.

When Mum comes with us in the car, it's up to me to make sure Dad doesn't get too angry. My duty is to protect her. It should be their job but I, the little one, feel that the responsibility rests on me. It's my task to make peace between them.

I remember clearly how Dad takes me to the Gröna Lund funfair to ride on a dodgem car. The other children swerve this way and that, colliding wildly and having fun. After all, that's the idea of the cars' thick, shock-absorbing rubber bumpers. But I have to drive around the edge nicely and carefully.

Collide? No, Svensson's daughters don't do that. I'm supposed to be practising for a driving test in the distant future — although I'm only 11 or 12 and we're in an amusement park where everyone else is having fun! It's Dad's views that govern everything — never my needs or wishes. My place is behind him. He may mean well, but he puts me under heavy pressure.

In interaction with the outside world, too, I learn to be quiet and not make demands. When the family arrive at a guesthouse on a road trip in France, I find that the sheets on my bed are very dirty. I want clean ones, but asking for such a thing is completely out of the question. Dad and Mum force me to sleep between disgusting sheets that some stranger has used. What I feel is totally irrelevant. The important thing is not to disturb the host couple. One mustn't be a nuisance...

Sneaky rebel

I feel invisible. I can't be truly visible because then they'd see me, Mum and Dad. Mum's like a little grey mouse apologising for its existence. Although I'm Dad's girl, he has extreme difficulty in understanding when I'm feeling bad. That feeling just doesn't exist.

Dad declares that he'll cut me out of his will if I take up smoking. So I smoke in secret. I smoke surreptitiously for years, from about the age of 11. It feels brave. The smoking is my little rebellion that he doesn't know about.

But I only dare to be a rebel in secret. Not once during my teens do I get home late in the evening. For my 15th birthday, I get a moped from my parents — in return for my promise that I'll behave. My friends know I always have to be the very first to go home.

About a year later, they divorce. Mum and Dad never talk to me about what's happening. I get no explanation for anything. There's just silence. Never, ever, do they say the divorce isn't because of me, that it isn't my fault.

Because I learn I'm such a pain to be with, it feels like it's me who messed things up for them. I should have saved our family. If I'd been good enough, they would have gone on living together, I think. It's a heavy responsibility. I keep my feelings bottled up.

Forbidden anger

Dad goes to live with his new woman, Barbara, in her apartment. On visits, I have to sleep in her sewing room, on an old wooden kitchen sofa that's far too short for me. I never get Dad to myself. It's always me, Dad, Barbara and her friends.

Barbara's adult children are often there too. This has been their home and, of course, they feel at home. For me, it's so obvious I'm just visiting — just kind of tagging along. No special arrangements are ever made for me and I don't feel welcome.

Being Dad's girl, I miss him a lot. Mum never encourages me to go and see him. She's so bitter. When I've been at Dad's place, she interrogates me about what we've done, whether his new woman has been with us and what she's said. I have to watch my tongue. I don't want to make Mum sad. The whole situation is fraught. She never, ever, asks how I feel.

In fact, I can't remember Mum ever asking how I was, or how I feel — not once during my whole childhood. Maybe she doesn't want to know. Maybe she doesn't know what to do with the answer if she asks something like that.

Dad and Barbara buy his parents' house. I think I'll be living with them there. Now there's space. Even when I'm 10, and feel that Mum and Dad will get divorced, I'm already beginning to fantasise that Dad and I'll move there together, to Gran and Grandpa's house. All these years, I've had a clear vision of it. I'm going to live in Grandpa's old phone room. I see it clearly ahead of me: my new room with the armchair, TV and carpet I've chosen myself.

I miss Dad and want to move there. Hope. Believe. But nothing happens. At last I ask plainly: 'Can I start planning what we're going to buy for my room?'

There's a deathly silence in the kitchen where we're sitting. The air hangs still between us. Dad keeps his mouth shut. Finally, Barbara blurts out: 'You must understand that you don't spend enough time with your Dad to get your own room. If you're going to live here, you'll be sharing a room with my weaving loom when you come.'

I feel completely cold, and go rigid. Everything feels so unreal. Dad does nothing to defend me. He lets Barbara decide. My rage burns inside and my heart is racing, but being angry isn't allowed.

Razorblade release

The question never comes up again. Throughout my childhood I have to learn, over and over again, not to be a nuisance. If I'm upset, it's just a matter of pulling myself together. Svensson's daughters never feel lousy. I don't argue. It just isn't done. But the clamped-down feeling of disappointment stays inside me, bottled up.

Not once do I sleep in their new home. My silent protest is to shun their house-warming party. If I can't live in that house, I don't want to go to the party either. Dad tries to persuade me, saying 'Sometimes you've actually got to do things you don't want to do.' But this time, in fact, I'm strong enough to defy his will.

I sense that Barbara's tired of teenage children. She's already coped with her own children through their teens, after all. She just wants Dad, not me, it seems. Mum's busy seeing her childhood sweetheart Alf and dealing with her own concerns. At home with her, I'm never allowed to mention Barbara's name. The lid stays on.

I'm extremely lonely. The knots in my stomach get worse. My throat tightens, panic creeps closer and I can't breathe. To hold back the anxiety and get the evil out of myself, I start cutting my body. I want to have a plaster cast on my arm — then my pain will show. I want everyone to see and understand. But it isn't possible.

All the time, I'm terribly sensitive to what others think of me. The worry about not being good enough is intense. When I imagine that others despise me, I have an overwhelming feeling of being a complete failure. I'm afraid of criticism. The idea of being rejected triggers my anxiety.

Chaos rules inside me, but can't be seen. Putting a brave face on takes a lot of effort. Even when I'm panicking, I manage to look happy.

Loneliness

Soon I meet a guy and fall in love. We get together. At 17, I have my life plan ready: by 25 I'll be engaged, by 26 married and by 27 a mother.

My boyfriend's mother wants to be a grandmother by the time she's 65. The demands are a tough challenge. I create my plan to avoid the nagging.

But the plan breaks down. After six years, when I'm 23, the relationship ends. At the same time, my girlfriends begin to have children. I've... failed.

When I tell my family I'm single again, a couple of months after he's moved out, Mum says: 'But Emma, why?'

I answer: 'I wasn't happy with him.'

Mum's comment — 'Well, is that so important?' — still hurts.

No one wonders how I feel or how my life is going. The only message I get is that being happy doesn't matter. I long so much for Mum to ask: 'Emma, how are you really?' But she never does.

It feels like Mum's biggest concern is, instead, that she feels under pressure to care for me now that I'm alone. She wants someone else to look after me, so she doesn't have to have a bad conscience. When I'm with my boyfriend and maybe go with him to his family's summer house in the archipelago, it's convenient for Mum to have me there, not at home. Then she doesn't have to care. Now when I tell her we've broken up, Mum's reaction is all about her own needs. 'Help, now I've got to look after Emma!' But the truth is, she's never had that responsibility. Mum's never taken care of me. Never, ever, has my mother looked after me.

I long for the kind of thing I think other daughters do with their mothers. I long for my mother to call and ask if I'll go to IKEA with her and look at curtains. That she'll say 'Hi, I need to go and buy shoes. Do you feel like joining me?' That she'll show, just once, that she wants to do something with me. But it never happens. Not once.

Betrayal

Again and again, I find that support from our parents is lacking. I swallow my disappointment, but finally something happens. It's the last straw.

My sister and I have long belonged to a football club, as both players and leaders. On one major anniversary, I get the honorary assignment of being the presenter, in front of 800 guests. It feels awesome. Full of joy and pride, I call Dad and say: 'You must come!' He promises to, but on the day he chooses to go to the theatre with Barbara instead.

Simmering with anger and disappointment, I call a crisis meeting at home with Mum. At 23, I finally put my foot down and confront Dad. 'I can't take this any more!' I say. A painful silence ensues. Mum and Dad squirm and say nothing.

I'm so awfully tired of other people's feelings always coming before mine. Like when it's my boyfriend's birthday and we have a party. On a day like that, I want both my parents there, but it's impossible. If I invite Dad, I have to invite Barbara too; otherwise, Dad won't come. But if I invite Barbara, Mum won't come. That's how it goes. Nobody cares that it upsets me.

That clinches it. Dad would rather go to the theatre with his partner than to the anniversary show that's so important to me. For seven years, he's chosen Barbara before me. Now I say, 'I want to see you without her.'

Finally, Mum and Dad look at each other and blurt out: 'We might as well tell you. We're moving back together. It's over with Barbara.'

My sister and I sit there, mouths gaping. Then we start laughing hysterically. It's so absurd. I can't believe they're serious, but they are. And once again, the focus shifts off me, my sadness and anger. I rise from my chair and stand there, unseen. I don't exist. Once again, I swallow the disappointment and go on being invisible. And the seven years Dad has spent living with another woman can never be mentioned again. They just vanish. It's all hushed up — again.

Self-punishment

For six years, I live alone. I feel inferior and increasingly unhappy, but I'm awfully good at keeping a poker face. If I see a girl with pretty fingernails on the Stockholm Metro, I go home and cry all evening. Alone. More and more often, I have destructive thoughts.

When I get sad, everything collapses. I'm never able to be a little sad. It's either fully on or off — shut-in feelings or a deep despair that totally takes over.

For a long time, I've wanted to end it all. It would be best for everyone if I no longer existed, I feel. I'm nothing like I should be. Life hasn't turned out the way it was supposed to.

When the panic comes creeping into my body, I think: Why do I have to feel so darn bad? Will it never end? I should feel well and be happy. A happy person doesn't feel like this. I shouldn't feel like this. I'm fine. Those thoughts give me a bad conscience where others are concerned, and make me feel even worse.

The anxiety is unbearable, but I show no sign of it. Secretly, I hurt myself. I shut my finger in the door on purpose. I cut myself with a piece of glass on the soles of my feet where it isn't visible and then, at work, stand all day long. I'm in constant pain, and feel I deserve it. It's frightening, but I really believe it.

Sometimes before going out shopping, I take both kinds of sleeping pill — to help me both go to sleep and stay asleep. Then I become totally unfeeling. It's dangerous, but I feel it's just what I deserve. Being already so weird, I think I might as well become even crazier.

Honesty

Finally, I seek help from a psychologist, hoping to get tools that will prevent me from getting so upset. It doesn't work. I go to several different therapists, but they just scratch the surface. I'm sick and tired of all the rating scales. No one gets to the bottom of my inner darkness. No one tries to reach into me, and I get new evidence that I don't really exist.

I sense that the therapists are alarmed by my suicidal tendencies. Keeping me alive, not understanding what it's actually about, is what matters most. And I'm ashamed of giving them such a hard time.

When I meet Erik, I'm struggling with a destructive self-image. At 29, I still place extremely high demands on myself. Daring to believe that he really wants to be my boyfriend is difficult. Because I'm taking masses of different tablets, it's hard to hide how things are going. Despite my skill in keeping a poker face, I now feel I have no room for secrets.

I decide to be completely open about my problems and tell Erik honestly about all my suicide attempts and medication. 'You must know this. Now you know what you have to decide about,' I say. Amazingly, he stays with me.

Erik understands that my mental problems aren't about him, and that they're due to my baggage from what I've been through previously in life. So he never says, 'Pull yourself together.' Instead, he supports me. What a huge difference from Dad, who just says, 'Forget it — just think about something else, and it'll pass.'

Hopelessness

Now I'm 38 and have long been treated for depression. I've had numerous rounds of various treatments, hospital admissions, sessions with psychologists and therapists… Twice, I've been in a psychiatric clinic and been given electric shocks (electroconvulsive therapy, ECT). The first time was 12 years ago.

My sister was seven months pregnant when I went into mental hospital. My anxiety was intense. At home, I'd broken a lot of glass, and cut myself on my arms and the soles of my feet. At the accident and emergency department, I thought they'd just bandage me up and give me a sedative, but I had to stay in hospital three weeks.

My sister was furious and said 'How the hell can you do this? You're going to be an aunt!' But I felt I just had to disappear. I wanted to spare her children from seeing me. I thought I'd come up with a clever solution: that if I died, her children would inherit my money.

When I was discharged, I had to show my face at the outpatient clinic every day. The suicidal thoughts were strong, so I wasn't allowed to have pills at home. Everything felt hopeless. After three weeks I was readmitted. This time, ECT was prescribed. I had 12 treatments.

It felt like I had no will of my own. I just longed to die. I got ECT so I wouldn't take my own life. I just remember the delightful feeling of being put to sleep. Not having to feel anything. Unfortunately, my memory gaps afterwards were terrible.

Once discharged, I was in touch with the outpatient clinic and various therapists, but felt they just scratched the surface. We talked about my upbringing, but no one understood that a whole lot of me was left behind in childhood — that I was kind of split into several parts.

Bottomless pit

At that stage in my life, I was sacked several times due to shortage of work. They were serious setbacks, but the diligent part of me applied for and got a new job every time. I struggled hard and worked full-time. After work, I would sleep for three hours. To free myself from the mental pain I scratched myself, bit my arm, cut my thighs and squeezed my fingers in a door.

It felt like I was spoiling life for everyone else. When I was at my worst, I tried to split up with Erik and break off friendships so that people wouldn't have to put up with me. The thought of slipping up petrified me. The slightest mistake shattered my self-image.

Spilling milk when I opened the carton might, I feared, have disastrous consequences. If I spill it, Erik won't like me any more. It means I'm a lousy daughter-in-law and he'll have to break up. The thought hit me in a flash and resulted in me not even daring to touch the carton — hardly even to exist. I felt simply terrible.

Five years after my first psychiatric hospital admission, I once more slid so deep into the murky pit of fatigue and depression that I was admitted again. The impulses to kill myself were powerful. It was important for me to explain to friends and, not least, work colleagues that I hadn't just hit the proverbial wall (which I saw as an 'in' phrase).

The whole of me felt as if I'd fallen into a great black hole. I had no will to get out again. How should I explain to wonderful Erik, who'd been in my life for over two years, that there was nothing for me to fight for? I genuinely wanted to die — just disappear and not struggle any more.

To relieve the anxiety, I cut myself again, this time on the soles of my feet. I felt totally worthless. I felt guilty about feeling so bad despite all the medication and therapy sessions I'd been given. I was so overwhelmingly tired of being sick. The anxiety was like a scream in my stomach.

Blunted

The ECT restarted. Then my boyfriend Erik put a stop to it. My memory wasn't working and he reacted strongly. By the time I asked for the fifth time on the same day how we'd met, he'd had enough...

The ECT was stopped after four treatments. Instead, I was given lithium, a drug that stabilises the mind and is used as an antidepressant when other treatment options have proved inadequate. Unfortunately, lithium can affect the thyroid gland so as to slow metabolism. It's common for people to put on weight.

I don't remember being informed about side-effect risks. It was just a matter of 'Open your mouth and swallow.' I put on 30 kilos and was unrecognisable. It was awful. With hindsight, through friends, I now realise it calmed and blunted me.

I have a long psychiatric history. Still, I've never cared what diagnoses the doctors have given me. It doesn't feel important. The medical records say 'major depression', 'personality disorder', 'borderline' and so on. I've been treated with CBT, DBT, dynamic therapy, ACT, ECT and lots of different medicines — antidepressants and anxiolytics, pills to induce and prolong sleep... I realise I need help, but all the time it feels like no one sees me. Nobody understands what it's like.

A war rages inside me. Feelings of guilt, shame, anger and grievance fight for my soul and sap my strength. Someone I know, aware of what I'm going through, tells me about the trauma therapist, TT. I send her an email, asking whether she can teach me to think differently, and she takes me on as a patient.

Several parts of me

I expect TT to show me how to make Dad stop saying stupid things. 'Tell me how to answer,' I ask. When I grasp that how I take what's said is what matters — that I can't, or don't need to, control others — it's a powerful revelation.

Together, we begin to explore what lies hidden beneath the surface. At first I'm very sceptical. I've already gone through so many treatments without them helping me. But soon I realise this therapy is helping me get in touch with what's been there in me all the time. It's right on target.

To start with, I don't see the patterns. I get overwhelmed by everything I encounter in the therapy. I have memory gaps and can't remember what we've discovered from one appointment to the next. But TT reminds me. I start to see connections. It's a long process that takes lots of energy.

Thoughts and feelings often pop up that don't seem to fit the situation or be in proportion to what's happened. Then the picture clears. I get in touch with several parts of me that seem to perceive events in completely different ways.

Now I know I have three Emmas inside me: Little Emma, aged five or six; Big Emma, the adult; and the teenager Dad's Girl. They think, feel and react in totally different ways and live at different times. It's amazing that we find them. Today, I find it hard to understand that I had no idea there were several of me. They were — and partly still are — so distinct, all three.

What makes me realise that several dissociative parts of my personality inhabit me is the answers that come when TT asks me something. I give a reply, but when she asks follow-up questions, I find that I don't always know what my reply has been — that it isn't me who chose to answer like that.

Then she begins asking 'Who said that? And who was the one who answered just now?' Sometimes it's Little Emma, sometimes Dad's Girl. I'm the same person all the time, but with several parts that have their own world view and different ideas about what's going to happen.

Internal fights

The therapy is an exciting journey into my inner self. We work intensively together, and the various parts of my personality begin emerging ever more clearly.

Big Emma is the one who goes to work, pays the rent and is diligent. On the surface she's good-looking, wears makeup and is strong. No one suspects that she wants to die because life isn't as it should have been.

Little Emma has many of the thoughts and opinions that don't fit into the adult world. She's the one who dreams of a fantasy Mum you go out, drink wine and eat prawn sandwiches with. The one who gets so incredibly sad when a friend or someone on TV says, 'My mother's my best friend.'

Dad's Girl is the hardest to get in touch with. She wants to be left alone. She deliberately makes herself alone to protect herself and be strong. She thinks therapy's nonsense. Of course, she gets very angry and upset when TT gets a look at her. At first, TT just gets to talk to her through the keyhole with the door closed. Dad's Girl doesn't want to let anyone in. 'Don't come here. Stop poking me!' she snaps. It's like picking on a scab and reopening the wound.

Dad's Girl, aged 16, is still living in her teenage days. On the surface, she's very cocky. She's a bit of a shrew. 'That's how to do it! That's not how to do it!' There are no nuances in her world. Everything's black or white.

Dad's Girl wants to live up to Dad's and Mum's expectations. She's prepared to do anything to make Dad like her, and she thinks he's always right when he says, 'Don't do anything we might be ashamed of.' She's well trained in knowing what's acceptable and what's forbidden.

This part of my personality has had great influence during most of my life. 'Don't stick out,' Dad's Girl yells at Big Emma. She keeps an eye on Little Emma, making sure she stays quiet and doesn't take up space. If you're not a particular kind of person, you might as well not exist at all.

Trapped in a dark room

Now I notice when the different parts appear and act. Dad's Girl is diligent and ingratiating. Dad's opinions govern her. She always wants to do the right thing and be obliging. Although I'm 38, this part remains a teenager. When Dad's Girl comes forward, I react and respond as if I were still there, at that time, in that state of dependence. The feeling that I shouldn't disturb people is very deep-seated. It's not good for me. Not healthy.

Dad's Girl is forever checking up on what's right and wrong. She's not allowed to take up space, as a mentally unstable person does. Showing off, or standing up for her own needs, provokes a feeling of shame. She goes with the flow. If I get angry with my partner and want to yell at him, then

Dad's Girl says 'Stop — you can't do that.' It's just a matter of pulling yourself together, she tells me.

She's trapped in a black room and doesn't even dare look out through the keyhole. At the same time, she has a strong will and wants to manage on her own. And she despises Little Emma — looks down on her because she's weak. From the start, she can't stand TT either. Dad's Girl thinks everything the therapist says is stupid.

Little Emma comes to the fore when I feel I mustn't be in the way. When I'm not allowed to press the button for the green man. Even today, in adulthood, I still find it hard to press that green-man button at the road crossing. I mustn't make life difficult for commercial drivers. If someone wants to get past me, I give way. I'd rather put myself in a tight corner than take up space. Today, my partner suffers from this.

Various strategies

I grew up believing that other people's needs are much more important than my own. Little Emma was brought up that way and still lives in those days. She's the six-year-old who wants to be good in Dad's eyes. She's extremely sure which rules apply. Little Emma thinks she's still living in Aspudden in her parental home, with Mum and Dad, but she doesn't live there any more.

Big Emma does everything expected of her. Dresses neatly and makes polite conversation. She's obedient and diligent. She'd rather jump through hoops than say no. However bad she feels, however little she slept last night, it would never cross her mind to turn up late for work or mess up an assignment.

Increasingly, during the journey, I've understood how my experiences have shaped me and how sharply divided I've become. When something happens in my adult life, it arouses strong feelings in me that originate from things that happened far earlier. The situation NOW triggers reactions from when I was little, without me knowing.

As a child, if I showed my sadness or anger I was rejected. The feeling of being helpless and abandoned was linked with shame. To protect myself, different parts of me have come up with various strategies to avoid that unbearable shame. Dad's Girl does everything right; she's a real know-it-all. Little Emma hides and becomes invisible. Big Emma pushes herself hard and is diligent.

The three parts of my personality are very angry with one another and often get into conflicts. There's a hell of a noise in there. Like a war. When Little Emma raises a question, Big Emma is there straightaway and suppresses her. Who do you think you are? Shut up! That's what it's like inside me.

Burning shame

Once when Erik and I visit a large building depot, we lose each other. Or, as I perceive it, I lose him. The situation of running around looking desperately for Erik sparks off a powerful flashback. Suddenly, Little Emma rockets back in time, straight into the vulnerability of childhood. It feels like she's lost Dad here and now. She's all alone and knows she's been told in the strictest terms to be obedient and not run around. Little Emma is scared, sad and desperate.

Dad's Girl is also thrown back in time, to her own reality. She's the one responsible for order. You mustn't lose each other. You must follow and keep an eye on your parent. Good God, what's she done now? That burning shame... all of it is imprinted so deeply in me. It's hard for Erik to understand what's happening inside me. He wonders why I'm so terribly beside myself. Why all the drama?

I see how crazy it is for me, aged 38, to have speech and reactions based, at different times, on a five-year-old's feelings, the world of a 16-year-old and an adult woman's values. The knowledge of my various parts helps both me and Erik to understand better what's happening in this kind of situation. He sees and talks to his adult partner. Suddenly he gets an odd reaction. Then it's reassuring to realise that it's Dad's diligent girl who's cut in, with her black-and-white values and her distinctive baggage.

Asleep in the hall

I contacted the therapist because I was so terribly tired. Where does my energy go? How can I be so exhausted that I barely have the strength to get home, close the door behind me and flop down in the hall? I'm completely convinced that TT will find and block the hole my energy is leaking out of. But there's no hole. The energy is there all the time, but I'm using it for completely the wrong things: it's fuelling my inner war.

Sometimes Erik finds me asleep on the hall floor with my shoes and jacket on. Then I feel like the world's worst partner. I'm horribly ashamed and think I might as well break up with him. I feel sorry for Erik, who has to spend time with me. That feeling sucks the life out of me even more.

Soon it becomes clear that I'm putting my energy into the wrong things. I can get worked up on someone else's behalf, but also beat myself up and bang my head on the radiator because I'm not good enough. I analyse and brood. Help, now Dad's said that. What does he mean by it?

I lack self-esteem. When I go on the Metro, it feels like everyone in the whole carriage is staring at me. What the hell's she doing here? How can she think she has the right to travel with us? That's what the destructive thoughts are like.

The loyalty to my parents is strong. I'm simply unable to act in any other way, despite all the feelings of inadequacy and shame I have to bear.

Since the day after I left school, I've had a job and behaved well. When I'm 23, I begin studying economics at university. I don't really know why. I have no dreams, no visions of what kind of job I want. 'You're so clever, you should really study,' I'm told.

I do well in my studies. All my exams go well. After a year of studying, I no longer want to go on. Why am I doing this? Do I need to study? Do I really want to study? Am I doing it for my own sake? Or just because everyone else is expecting it?

All my fault

The situation feels hopeless. I drop out of my studies and start working. Only after a month do I tell Dad and Mum I'm no longer studying. I know they'll have strong opinions about the decision, and I feel I need to be alone.

When I proudly tell Dad and Mum I've got a job as a secretary to a CEO, I expect them to be proud and happy. But they react negatively, asking, 'How on earth will you manage that?'

I've always felt that Mum and Dad are ashamed of me. They're disparaging when I get a new job. 'You change jobs like others change their underpants,' Mum comments contemptuously. I'm supposed to be nice and quiet. Not to grab. Not to develop. When things go well in my working life, they're ashamed because I get such a high salary.

One day, Mum comes to visit me at my workplace. To my boss she says, 'Can Emma really manage this?' I'm so used to her not believing in me that I don't react. But my boss does. After Mum leaves, the boss talks to me about what Mum has said. She would never say that about her own child, she declares.

I transfer my feeling of not being good enough to other people, too. If I ever invite my friends to my home, I can't enjoy their visit. I'm convinced they don't really want to come, but just don't know how to say no.

When I'm in hospital after a suicide attempt, my colleagues send a lovely bouquet. I feel very bad about those flowers. I keep thinking that they've wasted their working time ordering flowers for me when they could have done something more worthwhile. I ask Erik to throw the bouquet away. I can't believe they've given me the flowers because they like and really care about me. I'm absolutely convinced that people just hang out with me because they have to.

My head keeps spinning with wholly convincing thoughts: I'm all wrong. Everything's my fault. How everyone feels is my responsibility.

Compassion awakens

The medicines blunt my feelings and I'm addicted to the feeling the pills give me. I fight tooth and nail to keep the medication. I'm immensely scared of how I'd feel without my pills.

When I start the therapeutic process with TT, I'm on full-time sick leave, and mostly lie at home and sleep. It's a great defeat for me not to be able to work and justify my existence.

The therapy teaches me to think differently and know my own worth. Now I know I'm not the weak one. It's my parents. And now that I'm not putting my energy into what people call 'silly things', I feel much better about myself. We work a lot on that old feeling of being unworthy — a thought pattern I've got very hung up on.

Sometimes in the past, I thought it was only the lucky ones who got to walk on the finest beach promenade in life. Now I know and feel I have just as much right as everyone else. And that girl on the Metro with the impeccable nails doesn't make me despair any more. I just think: Okay, yes, it looks good, but I don't know how she feels under the surface. Maybe she's having a divorce. Or she might have cancer. After all, we know so little about each other. How we feel inside is invisible on the outside. I think about that every day.

Between therapy sessions, I do exercises at home. That reinforces the therapy. I read books borrowed from TT and listen to her words — the mindfulness exercises and compassion training she has adapted for me and recorded. A bit later on, I'm able to use apps about compassion that other people can also download. At first, putting myself first feels shameful, but I learn to be kind to myself. Step by step, I stop quarrelling with myself.

Several times a day, I can find myself reflecting on how I'm thinking and reacting now, compared with in the past. It strikes me that — wow! — if such and such had happened to me two years ago, I would have automatically thought I was stupid, and felt worthless. I used to punish myself for all kinds of things. Now I know it just makes things worse to put myself down. That's over now. I know my worth.

Medication-free

I may still sometimes think Erik and my parents would be better off without me, but I don't act out that feeling. Now I know it passes, and don't react so intensely any more. I'm learning to moderate my sadness when something bad happens. I don't tip over, and no longer fall into the black hole of despair and self-contempt.

Just over a year ago, it felt as if I had the lithium pills to thank for being alive. Lithium was my comfort blanket. I thought I'd be much worse off if I stopped taking the pills, but that wasn't true.

Today, I no longer need them and am infinitely proud and grateful that I dared let go of the medicine. I've gone from six tablets daily to zero without getting worse. I feel incredibly much better now. What a huge difference!

I can manage without the medicines I took for 15 years. Most people go on taking lithium throughout their lives. The fact that I could become completely medication-free is amazing! It's the therapy that has helped me. Lithium would never have given me the insights I've gained during the therapeutic process. Now I can even cope without antidepressants, which pleases me enormously.

At last I'm managing to shed my lithium kilos. Letting go of one kilo after another is liberating.

Heading for wholeness

The war's over. Step by step, Big Emma, Little Emma and Dad's Girl have come closer to one another. The various parts of me are getting on better. Each one knows about the others. They sit in a circle. Hold hands. Listen to one another.

When I say something spontaneously, I realise: That was Little Emma talking. And that was Dad's Girl. It's awesome. I'm working on understanding which one is active even before I speak. I'm getting completely, fully integrated. It makes a huge difference. Split into parts, I'm powerless. When they're joined together, I become powerful.

I realise it may sound vague and weird, like something made up, having several separate parts of your personality inside you. People fend off the truth and don't want to hear about it. But, for me, getting to know my parts has had a tremendously healing effect. I feel very strongly that there are three of us, that we belong together and have time to breathe. It feels quite all right for Little Emma to be small, as long as she can exist and occupy space. And the closer the parts get to one another, the easier it is to let go of the kinds of thing that make me feel bad.

The process of getting the parts of my personality to accept one another hasn't been easy. Dad's Girl, in particular, has been tremendously sceptical about approaching the others. She's been angry — furious, in fact! She's not at all keen on venting her rage against Mum and Dad. You don't badmouth your parents! But gradually she's realised that life's easier if we cooperate.

It feels good to be able to gather all the parts together when I want. Little Emma sits comfortably on Dad's Girl's lap. Big Emma and Dad's Girl are getting closer and closer. They hold hands and show great understanding of each other. For 90 to 95 per cent of my waking hours, I perceive myself as ONE person. That's great. They say and think the same things. But when things get a bit more strained, they sometimes separate again, disagree and want to do different things. It still doesn't feel quite natural for them to like one another in every situation.

The next step is to get all the parts working together automatically, with no effort.

Small advances

It feels like I've recaptured myself, bit by bit. Before, feelings governed my actions. Now I don't act out strong feelings directly, because I know they ebb away and pass. Difficult situations arise almost as often as before, but now I don't have to be overpowered by them. I can even laugh at them sometimes.

When life feels hard going, I'm no longer seized by panic. Instead, I go and lie down. Not to take refuge in sleep, but to look after myself when I've run out of energy. Both Erik and I know it passes. Knowing I will, in fact, recover is a great solace to us.

I'm immensely grateful for Erik's patience and love. He's had a very hard time and sometimes, I know, had his doubts. The hardest times have probably been when I've been convinced he would have been better off without me. When I've decided how he should think and feel. Thank goodness, Erik's a calm person. He sees that I'm making progress and understands that the healing process is slow.

We don't want to have kids. We've let go of that idea. Before, it felt like I had to give my parents grandchildren, but they've already got two thanks to my sister. Creating distance between me and my parents has been important.

Being an aunt to two children and godmother to another feels wonderful. I encourage them to venture to live their lives without thoughts that cramp their style. I'd cut off my right hand for them, and I say: 'You can do whatever you want. Fall in love with an Eskimo and move to Greenland if it feels right. The only difference it would make is that I'd get to travel to Greenland more often!'

No longer a victim

My parents show no interest in my healing process. Perhaps they see the therapy as a threat? Dad turns a blind eye. He says things like, 'Good God, are you still going there? You could talk to me instead, for free.' Mum wants to know what we talk about. 'Do you talk about me? About Dad?' She's worried for her own sake, not about how I feel. She doesn't seem to care that the therapy's making progress.

Obviously, I long for them to really care about how I feel and how the therapy's going. Still, I might have got suspicious if they'd suddenly become interested in my healing.

Therapy didn't work for Mum. Her truth is that therapy is a waste of money.

Mum was envious of the closeness between Dad and me when I was a child, and the envy still seems to be there. When I call Dad and talk for a while, he ends the conversation by reminding me of what I already know: 'Don't tell Mum that we talked. She gets so envious, you know.'

I'd really like to go for a long walk with Dad, just us two, but it's impossible. We never hang out, just him and me. On the contrary: Dad asks me to mediate and spend time with Mum, so that the situation stabilises.

I practise taking responsibility for my own feelings and situation. At the same time, I'm starting to make demands on others. Mum does her martyr act, saying it's Dad's fault she never travels or goes to the theatre. 'We never do anything nice. Dad doesn't want to,' she complains. The victim mentality has always suited her. Now that I've become stronger I say, 'Book tickets yourself, then!' instead of feeling sorry for her and guilty.

From shame to freedom

One theme of my new life is holding on to what's really important to me, and being loyal to myself. How I feel is important. It's very important for Erik and me to do well. Mum's problems are not that important in my life. Her needs aren't my responsibility. I can see it clearly, but the feeling is still split in two. Half of me cheers when I manage to let go of responsibility for Mum, but the other half still feels that pang of guilt.

My biggest fear is of becoming like Mum — a victim, with no self-esteem. The therapeutic process takes me ever further away from that path. Deep in my bones, I still feel the inhibiting message of never doing anything my parents could be ashamed of. But these days I'm going my own way. From shame to freedom.

I practise resting. Taking it easy is a new experience for me. An expert in taking care of others, I usually bend over backwards so that everyone else has a good time. It feels like my responsibility to get my group of friends together for a barbecue night, just as it was up to me to make sure our family got on well.

Investing energy in myself is new and very difficult.

Here's what a Saturday used to be like. Meeting a friend in the stable at eight in the morning to look after her children for a couple of hours while she went riding. Then making a beeline for another friend's place to babysit for a few hours so they can work on extending their house. After a quick snack at another friend's place, finding time for shopping, cleaning and preparing dinner for friends.

Now things have changed. The adjustment hasn't been easy. My friends mean a lot to me and I have to bite my tongue not to call and offer to babysit for them. Dad's Girl thinks I should take care of their little ones, now that I don't have any of my own — that it's expected of me. Now I've learnt that's my own expectation because I was brought up to be diligent. I'm starting to understand why I should take care of myself. That it's not mean to devote that energy to myself and Erik.

Little Emma's joy

Having your own opinions is wonderful. Still, it feels very new that I, Emma, can think something out for myself without talking to Dad first. What a difference!

My trauma is that Dad and Mum have turned a blind eye to me. They haven't seen what I've needed. You might think that's not too bad, but being invisible and neglected is like not existing. Not being there. Never getting your perceptions affirmed, never being helped to understand and manage how you feel.

My parents were emotionally inaccessible. They should have protected me, but I was the one who had to protect them instead. Still, I wasn't good enough. That realisation stung. I had to carry lots of guilt. Felt wrong. Bad. The shame limited me — made me weak. Eventually I felt completely worthless.

I am who I am because I was forced to learn how to survive as a child. I don't want to be ashamed of that. Now I'm stronger and act differently. It obviously affects other people. No longer doing what I 'should' arouses the sense of guilt. Dad's Girl protests wildly. But Little Emma revels in the freedom, drives around in the bumper car and has fun!

Acceptance

Throughout my life, I've longed for a mother who cares about me. One who calls and says 'Hi, how are you? Let's meet up, just you and me, shall we?' A mother who shows warmth. The therapy has helped me understand I'll never have a mother like that — she exists only in my imagination. When I realise that, I scream out loud with disappointment.

Now the therapist and I have laid my dream mother to rest. Symbolically. I drew all the maternal love I had fantasised about, and then buried that much-longed-for love. It was painful, but at the same time delightful to finally let go. I mourn for the mother I've never had, and feel free.

A powerful moment in the therapy lingers on. It's the moment that makes me dare to take a decisive step out of the shame and into freedom. I've always wanted to play drums. We talk a lot about it. Finally, TT arranges for us to go to a rehearsal studio where some young guys often play rock music. I get to sit by the drums, and she encourages me to play. Oh, I want to so much! But am I really allowed to have a go at the drums? Make a noise?

The voice inside me says, 'NO. You'll disturb the neighbours. They'll get angry, and come and complain. Then you'll be ashamed.' But I'm so keen to try.

I have to check everything. Is the room soundproofed? How thick is the door? How far is it to the neighbours? Then I defy that voice that belittled me. I drum wildly. It feels superb. What a victory!

Well at last

I can't really remember when I last noticed that one of the dissociative parts of my personality was active. One day when I'm sitting with TT, we try to contact them as usual. Usually I sense them, but now I can't find them. Little Emma, Dad's Girl, Big Emma... they simply aren't there any more!

I feel good inside and it shows. People around me notice the change and say, 'Welcome back!' When I was least well and in the mental hospital, I put on lots of weight, and it stayed for many years. In the past, I didn't think I could cope without the medicine. I used to say, 'Don't touch my lithium!' But I proved able to cope.

Step by step, I've struggled to recapture my body. To date, 28 of the 30 excess kilos have disappeared. My successful weight loss makes me feel incredibly good and proud. It's awesome to look, again, like I did 10 years ago and be able to move so easily.

Neither did I think I could cope without support from TT. No way did I want to let go of that sense of security. Don't touch my therapist! It felt like that, very strongly. I was afraid of falling back into old patterns. But the fear has gone. I trust TT to know what she's doing. She would never encourage me to let go of the medicines or the therapy if she weren't convinced that I'd manage it. She doesn't take chances like that.

Now we've phased out the sessions and completed the therapy. It feels good. I'm standing on my own two feet and feel completely well. Getting sad sometimes isn't that bad. I can sort out my feelings and reflect with some perspective. In the past, when my personality was in three parts, each reacted in her own way. It was confusing. Now that I'm a whole person, I can more easily sort things out by asking myself, What's this about? Why do I react as I do? What can I do to create a good outcome?

I'm free

At work, I'm tested every day in various situations, but now I'm confident and say no when it gets too much. The firm I work at has been taken over by another company and major changes are coming, but I'm not worried. Instead, I see new opportunities opening. Woohoo, I'll get 60 new colleagues!

In my private life, too, I keep tabs on my limits. I make sure to look after myself and recover. Rest isn't a bad thing. It's good! And I trust that other people are fully capable of taking care of themselves. They aren't my responsibility.

I'm no longer angry about Mum being as she is, not reacting or behaving as I want her to. I often think of the moment when I symbolically buried my dream mother under a pillow and laid flowers on the grave. That ritual really helped me to let go and block the hole where my energy was running out.

Three parts have become one. I am myself: Emma. It's a wonderful feeling. The memory of the experiences that held me back is still there, but no longer controls me.

This summer, Erik and I are getting married. My desire has awakened. We're living here and now. Life's good. I'm whole. I'm free.

CHAPTER 7

Attachment system: the necessary bonds

Children's need for attachment is as basic as their food and warmth requirements. A broad definition of trauma usually also includes 'attachment trauma'.

At birth, we are totally dependent on others. We are equipped to survive, and need the group we are born into. Closeness to and good companionship with others are essential. The care that adults provide and our interaction with our first caregivers shape us, laying the foundation for our contact with others. Without lasting emotional intimacy, we cannot develop into fully functioning adults.

Our experience of relationships during those vital early years, in particular, creates patterns that determine how we deal with difficulties and get on with others. These 'attachment patterns' persist into adulthood and influence us, especially in all our close relationships. They become a kind of inner working template that we follow without seeing it ourselves.

Almost all of us are born with a basic capacity to receive and give care. This may be said to be the basis for our ability to feel deep compassion for others and ourselves. We can therefore realise, feel and understand another person's perspective and want to help if someone else is suffering. We carry this inner ability through life, but it can also be trained and get the chance to grow and become more accessible.

Will to live

We cannot choose the circumstances we are born into. Much can happen and we do our best to cope, feel happiness and joy, and have a meaningful life. This is fundamental and applies to every child, whether fortunate or disadvantaged and regardless of whether our custodians are good enough, inadequate or perhaps even dangerous for us.

We are born in complete dependence, with strong instincts to seek care and protection from the adults closest to us. When we are hungry, tired, in pain and, for example, sad or frightened, we automatically turn to our caregivers — first, to understand what is happening and, second, to get help in regulating our feelings about the experience.

But how can we understand that, as adults too, we often react and do things that are incongruent with how we really want to behave? The will is not the only thing that governs us. We are biopsychosocial beings. The human body is programmed for survival, and must have a brain directing how we use our physical abilities, but we cannot cope without belonging to social contexts. Our interplay with the surroundings we are born into, and develop and live in, is constant. None of these three factors — brain, body and social context — is dispensable. We cannot manage without them.

Lightning reactions

We are prepared both for a life in security and for trying to survive threatening situations. Our inherited systems react to what we experience. These reactions come automatically, without our becoming aware of them. We can all feel shame, terror, rage and so on. Sometimes our reactions are prompted by the wish to rid ourselves of the very emotion we feel; since we perceive it unconsciously, we do not always understand ourselves. We all react automatically with the impulsive urge to get rid of the negative emotional states. Sometimes we resort to action, giving vent to rage, before we can stop ourselves.

Some of the negative emotions we seek to reject are strongly associated with the threat system. On the other hand, we want more of the positive emotions like joy, the curiosity and the urge to strive for closeness and love. These we want to keep, certainly not let them end — sometimes, so much that we do not even enjoy the positive emotional times because we think they will soon nonetheless end. Several of these positive emotional states are firmly connected with the attachment system.

Importance of security

From birth, we experience what being with others is like. If we are treated with compassion, we expect compassionate treatment to usually be forthcoming later. The same applies to being understood, seen and treated with warmth, friendliness and respect. Our life experience tells us, *This is what being with others is usually like.*

With well-functioning interaction during the key first years of life, we get help from our attachment persons in coping with our experience of anxiety and fear. When we need protection it is given, and we learn how to deal unaided with our painful feelings as well, and control them. Our early experience then gives us a robust basic pattern of faith in ourselves and others, and this is the perspective from which we understand the world. We develop security and trust.

Trusting individuals get a capacity for balanced closeness to and distance from other people, and develop their innate ability for compassion and will to help themselves and others. We can regulate our feelings and emotional states, manage our perceptions and express our emotions in a balanced way. We are able to express our needs; we can say yes to things, but also say no to what we do not want. We are capable of standing up for ourselves. We can do this without anguish and without worrying about not being liked. Our emotional regulation is intact and works well.

Infants' emotional reactions to separation from, and breaks in interaction with, their caregivers have long been studied, and the theory of attachment and attachment patterns has been created. Research has given us extensive knowledge of the importance of basic security and the consequences of its absence in early childhood, particularly during our very first year of life. Today, this is a highly influential theory that emphasises the importance of closeness and love in our lives.

Patterns can change

We are often unaware of the attachment patterns that are imprinted in us, affecting our relationships. We are born with a spectrum of unconscious biological 'affects' (emotions, or strong feelings). Assisted by our parents or other caregivers, we necessarily learn to regulate our emotions.

The association between mental suffering and illness in adulthood is strongly linked to our attachment patterns. Studies show that chaotic (commonly known as disorganised) attachment patterns are more than twice as common in people who need psychiatric help in adulthood than in those who never consult a psychiatrist. These patterns apply to both physical separations and disruptions in mental communication. Being rejected or neglected generates anxiety, fear, confusion, uncertainty, insecurity and self-accusations.

Understandably, neglect, humiliation and denigration shape what children think about themselves. They affect infants' cognitive, as well as neurobiological development. Children then construct internal negative models and patterns of thoughts like *I'm bad, I'm helpless* and *I'm hopeless*. As a result, other people or external circumstances will govern their lives. Positive self-perceptions are interpreted as distortions of reality. This increases the risk of developing complex post-traumatic stress disorder (PTSD), making the vulnerability factor high.

It is above all in new situations and in interactions with people close to us that these patterns we have created are revealed. Are we able to soothe ourselves, balance closeness and distance in relation to others, and withstand times of sadness or fear? Can we manage all this, or does it awaken unconscious reaction patterns in us that are based on past insecurity?

If no profound psychological work is done, our attachment patterns persist throughout life. Fortunately, they can change. We can acquire secure attachment by various means, including psychotherapy. As noted earlier, the brain is more plastic than was previously believed.

Four attachment patterns

Four categories of attachment pattern are commonly recognised:

- secure
- insecure-avoidant
- insecure-ambivalent
- disorganised (or disoriented).

People with the secure attachment pattern have sufficiently good trust in themselves and the outside world. Children with this pattern have a sound, moderate degree of caution towards strangers. They have no major difficulties in getting used to the presence of a playmate's parent, turn to this person when they need help, and expect to get it in a friendly way and as a matter of course.

With either of the insecure attachment patterns ('insecure-avoidant' or 'insecure-ambivalent'), a person often manages to live close to others in adulthood, albeit with some difficulties. Avoidant and ambivalent attachment patterns make a relatively fragile foundation. They cause greater vulnerability than the secure attachment pattern. Nonetheless, people with insecure patterns have nowhere near such big difficulties in close relationships as those with a disorganised attachment pattern.

Insecure attachment

These patterns are unconscious and automatic. We do not choose them. Children with an avoidant attachment pattern have had caregivers who have failed to meet –the children's needs for closeness in a balanced, secure way. The caregivers have not been able to help them regulate their emotions in the way, or to the extent, that these children needed. The adult may have reacted dismissively, or failed to see and understand the child. Sometimes the adult may even have punished and frightened the child. These children have learnt to suppress and hide their longing for closeness, withdraw and not seek contact or support. Experiencing many situations in which support and close contact with others have not been forthcoming creates lonely children who easily succumb to recurrent thoughts about themselves as bad, inadequate or inept and inferior to others.

Children with an ambivalent attachment pattern have received care from their caregivers that has been capricious and unpredictable. The adult has sometimes been responsive and helpful, but at other times dismissive, negligent and even hurtful. The parents may have been engulfed in their own feelings and unable to see the situations from their children's point of view at all.

Owing to these two insecure attachment patterns, relationships in adulthood can become problematic. No serious psychological problems necessarily exist in adulthood, but the unconscious patterns are automatically activated in close, intimate relationships. They often create problems in couple relationships and when people form their own families.

Chaotic attachment

A totally chaotic attachment pattern is usually termed 'disorganised'. Children with this pattern have experienced horrifying situations in relation to their caregivers and have had to seek care and closeness from the very individuals who directly harmed them with violence and abuse or neglect. To survive, these children have had to try repeatedly to get help from people who hurt them in one or more ways. Children never know how to deal with this situation. *Will I be abandoned or attacked?* The little individuals never know what will happen next, and try to ward off the harm to the best of their ability. The world and other people are perceived as dangerous.

To survive, children need to form attachments. This is a strong, fundamental instinct. The ties of attachment do not weaken even if children face violence. They are utterly at their caregivers' mercy, in an experiential world of horror, abandonment and chaos. They have no chance of regulating their own perceptions, feelings and behaviour, or their surroundings.

If, while growing up, we suffer from ever-recurrent traumatising experiences, and have no secure attachment person, there is thus a major risk of our developing a 'disorganised attachment pattern'. The strategies that children can develop to survive are many and resourceful, but they are always created at the expense of the children themselves and their existence. In adulthood, people with this kind of attachment pattern often have difficulties in relationships generally, rather than just intimate, close ones. Living with truly serious attachment trauma is the same as living with a disorganised attachment pattern.

The infant's inner world

As healthy newborn babies, we are totally absorbed in our own perceptions. We do not connect what we experience with who we are, what has just happened or what will happen in the future. Our various needs are regulated in a range of behavioural systems. We shift among various emotional states and have no unitary sense of self.

Even if infants could speak, they would be unable to describe their perceptions coherently, so that others understand what they mean. They would still lack the ability to understand the world on the basis of a self, let alone express this intelligibly. There would be no consistent message in their communication. Their shifting feelings are sharply distinct from one other and their behaviour is regulated by needs and emotions. If we could relive our infancy from an ordinary adult perspective, we would probably perceive that existence as fragmented.

This is entirely normal and healthy for a baby, but as we grow we need help in connecting our perceptions, creating inner structure and becoming a cohesive personality. In this process, we need caregivers who affirm our feelings and experience, enabling us to connect inner perceptions with external events. This imparts context to our existence: the past, present and future, and what we see, hear, taste, feel, think; and the connections among them (sensory-motor coupling).

Imprinted patterns

In the first few years of life, we successively acquire ever more experience. We connect our perceptions and, if we feel secure, we develop an ability to perceive ourselves as individuals. We understand that someone who is not in our field of vision can still exist as a person. *Mum exists, even when I can't see her.* And: *The person in the mirror is me.* A little later, we realise that other people have their own feelings and thoughts.

Children seek security to get help in coping with painful feelings, such as fear. In an unfamiliar situation, they look for the adults on whom they depend. If the adult's behaviour affords no sense of security and, instead, is strange and frightening in terms of the child's situation, the result is a dilemma for the child.

If the person a small child is dependent on cannot provide the security and calm the child needs, the foundation of the insecure attachment pattern is laid. The child's solution might be to gain protection through avoidance — perhaps by escaping inwards, for example. Taking refuge in oneself, or fleeing from contact, is a dominant feature of the avoidant attachment pattern.

Ambivalent attachment means that children sometimes try to resolve the insecure interaction by means of distance, but sometimes with exaggerated closeness, for example in the form of clinging.

Thus, disorganised attachment is the most severe aberration. For such children, interaction with their caregivers is erratic. They are unable to create enduringly secure patterns in their behaviour with others. The pattern becomes chaotic and devoid of trust.

Drops eroding stone

To lower the number of people with post-traumatic stress disorder (PTSD) and dissociation, is to reduce the family violence and abuse that occur in homes and close relationships. Children subjected to this mistreatment at home are at constant risk. The stories below in this book show how the family home becomes a minefield, where one never knows what will happen next. Constant vigilance is the rule. At any moment, getting out of harm's way may be necessary. This unpredictability imposes intense, continual stress. For growing children this is even more devastating, and strongly affects their development. The earlier in life the children are affected, the worse the consequences. If the people subjecting children to traumatic experiences are the attachment persons themselves, on whom the children are dependent, the consequences are even graver.

What, then, happens when children suffer violence and abuse? What is the outcome if the mistreatment is repeated over and over again, and the relationships are never repaired? What if, perhaps, the perpetrators also deny or make light of what has happened, claim the role of victim for themselves or blame the children for the course of events? What if perpetrators frighten children into silence? And if family members, neighbours, professionals and the community at large are reluctant to either see or hear about what is going on?

In a growing child, the parts of the brain that receive most stimulation are those that develop most. A secure existence activates curiosity, play and imagination. Fear activates and develops the threat system instead. Then, the internal alarm goes off. The child must be poised for self-defence at any moment. Every sense is strained to the limit.

How can anyone live a harmonious life under such circumstances, or afterwards?

Drops erode stone not by their weight, but by falling incessantly.

SECOND STORY

As adults, we can lead a life with enough security to function relatively well from day to day. But suddenly something unpredictably dreadful, perhaps an infinitely painful loss, throws us into an acute crisis that immediately gets our threat system going. *How can I protect myself? How can I survive this? It can't be true... is this really happening?*

Step by step, we must take in the disaster we have suffered. We need time, and sometimes help. Our internal stability may not be quite sufficient. To resolve the crisis, we then have to fall back on strategies we have unconsciously used before — the kinds that do us no good in the long run. This occurs automatically. It is what being human involves.

No doubt we all know the feeling of wanting to escape from something we are experiencing. Sometimes we avoid specific experiences too intensively, for too long. Somewhere, surely, we know this but are not quite able to break the pattern.

Christine did not want to be like a robot any more. Going around as if in a bubble and not feeling anything at all is terrible, she told TT when she phoned.

Christina Lejonöga : Annica Lilja Ljung

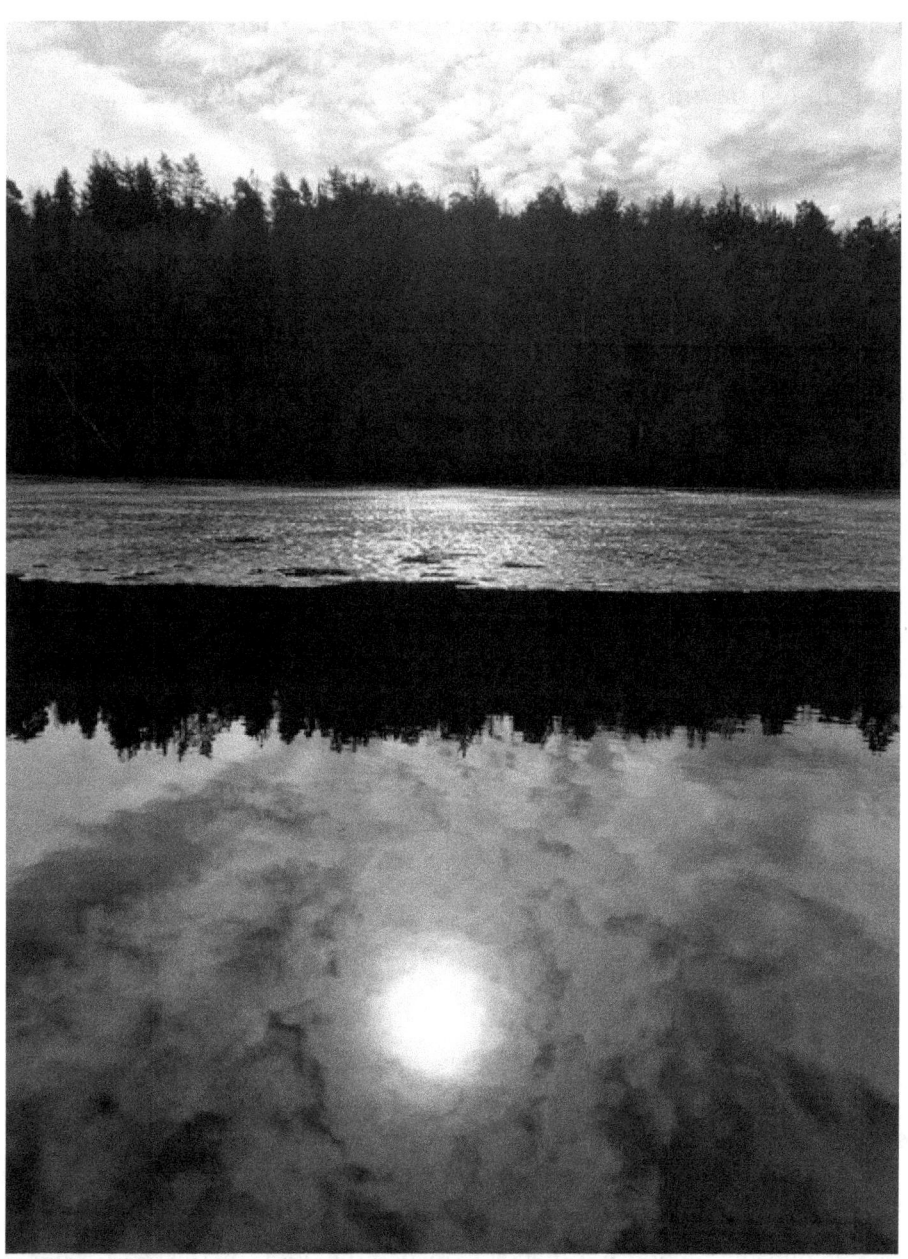

By *Elina Ehn*

Christine

Christine loses her son in an accident. What matters most in her life is gone. The shock makes her switch off her feelings completely. Instead of grieving and moving forward in life, her heart remains mute.

'Suddenly, death snatches away my beloved child. My entire future with him just vanishes. I'm shut inside a bubble of locked feelings.'

One rainy Tuesday in October, 14 years ago, my life totally changes direction.

I'm married, with two wonderful teenage children and a job I enjoy. Life is going tremendously well. That day, straight after work, I go to the shop next door, where my son John works. I decide to drop in and say hi.

But John isn't there. He hasn't shown up yet.

I'm not worried. I know John can look after himself. He's 19 years old and due to leave school in the spring. He's a bit tired of studying, admittedly, but in the last year at upper secondary school he's far from the only one. He has a nice girlfriend and a part-time job at the shop, and is about to get both a flat and a permanent job. I'm pleased, and proud of our son.

Arriving home, I don't see his car in the car park. Strange. *Could I have overtaken him on the road?* When I open the front door, I hear my daughter crying. I rush into the living room and see her sitting there on the sofa, tears running down her cheeks. Two adult strangers are there too. A chill comes over me.

The unimaginable

'We have something sad to tell you,' says one police officer. *'Your son is dead.'* I stand there in the middle of the floor, as if in a bubble. Time stands still. I feel as if I'm going to faint. They help me to the sofa and I lie there limply, without understanding. It can't be true. It must be a mistake.

But reality presses in. I'm told that Amanda, our 15-year-old, saw the two people outside the house. When she opened the door, they asked for her parents. Neither of us were at home. Then they told Amanda her brother was dead.

John's car aquaplaned and collided with a lorry. *'We've been recommended to tell you that you shouldn't see him,'* the police officers say. My mouth says I understand. But everything feels empty. I can't take it in. I don't scream. It's like I'm not there. When my husband George comes home, the police say, *'You'll cope well with this,'* and left us.

Robot-like, I ring our closest relatives and tell them John is dead. I hear other people's reactions, and it's as if I've stepped out of myself. After I've talked to my father, it doesn't take many minutes for my mother to call. *'I don't understand why you had to be in such a hurry to buy a car for him,'* she says. The room goes dark and the floor falls away from under my feet. Instead of uttering a few comforting words, she lays all the blame on us. It's a heavy burden. I wish Mum had said, *'Oh how sad,'* and come here and hugged me.

Up here in my brain I grasp the fact of John's death, but not in my heart. Common sense tells me the accident is neither my fault nor my husband's. We had reasoned so intelligently that it was better to buy a good car with new winter tyres for our son than for him to drive around in borrowed vehicles we knew nothing about. John was a cautious driver. He had a good car. It was drizzling. The conditions caused aquaplaning; it was just bad luck. *The accident can't be my fault...* Still, the sense of guilt pierces deep inside me.

Brief farewell

At five o'clock the next morning, the doorbell rings. I get up and spontaneously think *Now John's coming!* My hopes are up. *Someone might have stolen his car... so someone else was behind the wheel of the crashed car, and the news of his death was an error...?* But it isn't John standing there in the hall. It's George's sister with her family. They have driven all night to be with us and share the grief.

We drive to the scene of the accident. The only signs of what has happened are a few pieces of metal left lying on the road. The police officers have told us the driver of the heavy goods vehicle did all he could to avoid the collision, but John crashed straight into it.

It feels grim to have no chance to say goodbye — not to see him or even stroke his hand one last time. My son is dead *and* taken from me. *How broken is he really?* In my mind's eye, I see horrifying cinematic images of bodies torn apart. I have to know. I phone the Forensic Medicine Department and am told it's the police who decide.

At the police station, we have a long wait. I have no sense of time, but recall lots of people coming and going, fetching their new passports and staring at us where we sat waiting. Finally, we get to meet a police officer, who gives us a brown bag with John's watch and a lot of beads from the necklace he always wears. The firefighters picked up all the beads they found at the accident site. Their thoughtfulness is touching. *Now I can rethread the necklace so that John can wear it for the burial.*

The police give us the go-ahead to bid farewell to John. Amanda, George, my brother and I go to Forensic Medicine, where the body is stored. There he lies, serene, with his eyes slightly open. His nose is a bit damaged. He has grazes on his forehead and a tooth is missing. But he's unbroken. The room is peaceful, with lighted candles and fine brick walls. I stroke John's hand, and kiss him. He's gone, I feel: it's just his cold shell lying there.

It's a brief farewell. I lack the presence of mind to say I want to bring a chair in and sit with him for a while. Nobody gives us any guidance or support. Afterwards, I feel very disappointed about being given the wrong information and advice from the police officers who told us of his death. They were unreliable. Robbed of a future with John, we nearly have to go without the final parting, too. How strong and demanding do you really have to be when you've lost your child and are in shock?

The accusation

The following day, the priest comes to our home. We talk about the funeral and she tells us about a funeral parlour that is open to the idea of playing John's favourite music instead of traditional organ music.

Flowers and greetings pour in. Every time the doorbell rings, it gives me a good feeling. All that consideration is kind. But all those flowers are driving my husband crazy. It's striking how differently we react. Many adults seem to be avoiding us, but John's friends are brave. In the midst of the shock, 18-year-old Daniel rings the doorbell, with a small plant, and asks, *'Hi, can I go into John's room for a while?'*

When the time comes to bury John, my mother can't resist doling out blame again. *'It's such a shame that John's brought this on us like this,'* she says, accusingly. I've lost my beloved son, but get no comfort from my mother, no guidance on how to manage one's grief.

The funeral is fine. The church is crowded and it's good to see how many people have come. I feel a little detached in there. My body shakes throughout the ceremony, but I can't cry. Suddenly the sun shines through the window, like a sign, and I feel a comforting hand on my shoulder.

In the evening, we have an open house for John's friends. The whole hall is full of shoes. How I've missed that since John disappeared — the piles of big shoes that we have to step over! Suddenly they're gone. Now, for a single evening, they're back again. We watch a film of John rock-climbing and I get a chance to see new sides of my son through his friends' stories. New, positive images, confirming his existence, appear. As long as we're talking about John, a small piece of him remains.

No breathing-space

I live as if in a vacuum. The day after the funeral is Amanda's birthday, and we celebrate it. Soon it's Christmas. Amanda wants everything to be as usual at our home. She wants to be a happy girl, despite everything. I've already bought a Christmas present for John. What should I do with it? And the Christmas cards — how can we send them? What shall we write? Having only three names on the card is unthinkable. It will have to be *Merry Christmas from the Ekberg family.*

John's death is a catastrophic loss. We receive help, of course, but it's only superficial. A deaconess comes to our home a couple of times, and a week after the tragedy I have to go to the health centre to register for sick leave. This results in us meeting a counsellor four times. George lets it out by speaking, putting what has happened into words, but we get no help in talking over how we can move on. The experience becomes frozen in place. I can't really understand what has happened to me. A thin scab grows over the wound, but it's still infected beneath.

Soon I'm back at my job. Working is considered best, obviously. You mustn't stay at home and mourn. When I stand there outside the school door, my pulse throbs. My heart is pounding. Now I'll come up against everyone's fear: that of my colleagues as well as the parents. *Oh, there she is — the one who lost her child.* I see the horror shining in their eyes.

Going back to work feels strange. Everyone means well, but of course I have to go back to the old routines. Being there for others. Being nice. As a teacher, you're needed by the children all the time. You have no time to yourself, no respite. My husband, a plumber, gets chances to talk about his grief while working. A workmate who has also lost his child helps him get through the loss. That opportunity doesn't exist for me.

Why can't I cry?

I try to work half-time but take no pleasure in being alive. After all, John is dead. I long to dream about him, but it takes ages to happen. Missing him is paralysing.

Sometimes people say stupid things. Once when I'm about to go home after half the working day, my colleague says, *'It's nice for you to be able to go home now.'* Her words hurt. Silently, I wonder whether she wants to swap places…

An acquaintance visits our home, sits there on the sofa and cries because his old aunt has died. No doubt he just wants to show solidarity, but it hurts inside me. I want to yell, *'Your children are alive — my son is dead!'* But I keep silent.

Time passes. I'm with the children, available to them at school, but my own gigantic loss is unreal. *What's wrong with me? Why can't I cry? Aren't I mourning properly?* My conscience has found another reason to plague me. But John whispers quietly inside me: *'Mum, I know you're grieving in your way. It's okay.'*

On the first anniversary of his death, I'm back at the scene of the accident. For perhaps ten minutes, I stand there in the dark at the roadside. Seeing it again, the place where John crashed, is a kind of confirmation that the unimaginable had really happened. Suddenly, a breakdown vehicle slows down. The driver, seeing me, has remembered the accident in the pouring rain the winter before. I'm touched that he takes the time to stop and talk.

New start

I continue working half-time. That's all I can cope with. My body is often extremely tense and I get palpitations and have to run to the bathroom. My whole being shakes as the panic creeps back. I've lost my son, but I've also lost the ability to be the mother I should be to our daughter. The threat of a new severe loss is constantly lying in wait, and makes itself felt again whenever anything reminds me of the trauma of John's death.

If Amanda has promised to be back home no later than ten in the evening but hasn't turned up by three minutes past, I begin planning her funeral at once. Anxiety and thoughts of disaster are sparked off immediately. If one of the children can be snatched away, then it can happen again.

Once a week for just over two years, I meet a psychologist. But I see through her strategies and give her the answers she wants, without letting her get close to me. Talking gives me momentary relief, but I get no tools for managing my inner life. So I forget about that — not because I want to, but because I can't express myself and the psychologist doesn't understand.

Four years after the accident, it's time for a change. Amanda has grown up and moved away from home. George and I sell the house and move north. A fresh start feels good and we're in the right place — one John loved. There, he played, swam, went fishing and camped out. We make a memorial in the garden with beautiful stones from the seashore. All summer, flowers grow in profusion there. In the winter, the grave lantern lights up John's place every evening.

In the village, I get in touch with a new therapist. We meet regularly for almost two years, but this time too I just go through the motions. He doesn't get inside my shell either. I make no progress.

Birth of hope

When the South-East Asian tsunami takes place, I'm deeply affected. Many parents lose their children in the flood waves. The newspapers and TV programmes are full of death and crisis management. When I read about the four phases of crisis — shock, reaction, processing and reorientation — I realise that even if it's supposed to be like that for everyone, it's not at all accurate for me. According to that book, I'm still in the shock phase: emotionally screened off, seemingly unaffected. I haven't cried, screamed or hurled things in despair. Since John's death, I've locked in everything I'm feeling. The thoughts have never been processed, and the grief has barely begun to heal.

In my quest for consolation, I read books about other people who had suffered trauma. It helps me a little. The turning point comes when I read about a mother who has lost her husband and two children in the tsunami. She talks about the experience of being shut inside a bubble of sealed-in feelings. On the outside, she looks the same as before, as if nothing has happened. Inside, she is marked by the pain that never seems to ease.

When the mother in the book puts those feelings into words, I recognise myself. Her description matches me so well. How has she moved on in her grief? Through Facebook, I get in touch with her, and she tells me she has received good support. She understands me and says I too need help. She thinks I should contact TT, and give me her phone number. True, I'm a bit bruised after my previous contacts with psychologists, but I really want to change my life. I can't go on like that — I've had enough.

Tears at last

Ever since John's death, I've been emotionally mute. Switched off. For 13 years, I've lived like a robot, with my own feelings out of reach. Finally, I call TT and we meet. I fill in rating scales and am interviewed. After assessing me, she says I had post-traumatic stress disorder.

TT says it may work for me to try something called EMDR. She explains in detail how it works. A therapeutic method based partly on eye movements — can that really work? I want to try.

At the next session, I have to first find a 'safe place' inside myself, and then answer some questions. We follow a manual. TT asks me to think of an episode. I choose an event after John's death, and fix all my attention on this memory while my gaze follows TT's fingers as they move back and forth. After a series of movements I have to stop, take a deep breath and take note of my thoughts and feelings. *'What do you feel in your body?'* she asks, and I answer. We go on working intensively: moving my eyes, resting, staying with the memories that appear. Slowly my feelings emerge, bit by bit — without me completely falling apart. Unbelievable!

My body reacts. Now the trembling starts. I feel a crying sensation in my throat. TT encourages me to stay in that feeling and keep exploring, ever more deeply, what's happening in me. My heart pumps wildly and the urge to cry grows into a giant lump in my throat. I'm someone who has never stopped to reflect before; I've avoided feeling; and struggled to shut it all in. But now I'm staying with my inner feelings and daring to open up. *What am I feeling?* The guilt hits me like a bolt of lightning, straight into the core of me. *It was my fault.* Rather than fleeing, I penetrate more deeply into my feelings. Instead of trying to understand my mother, and defending her because she doesn't know better, I allow myself to experience *my own* feelings.

The pain and grief are overwhelming. At last I can cry. I lie on TT's floor and weep out all the pent-up despair. When I allow myself to really experience the feeling, I notice that it finally releases its grip on me and goes away. The blockages dissolve. I have no guilt. It's like magic!

Insights

That intense experience during the treatment marks the beginning of an inner journey. In a secure context, I venture to feel the dark pain that the grief work requires me to get through. At last I can move on. After my liberation in the therapy room, I'm able to cry at home when I need to. It feels wonderful.

It's great to *feel* — that I finally *can* feel. Now that I'm in safe hands, yelling and sobbing no longer feels dangerous. Past therapists have just talked to my reason and told me, *'Go home and cry.'* They have never helped me feel, or cry. Now I'm learning both to feel and cope with my feelings.

John's death has brought my life to a head. Although the trauma took place many years ago, it has affected my daily life through post-traumatic symptoms like emotional shutdown, and other obstacles to leading a good life. Everyone has patted me on the back and said, *'Christine, you're so strong!'* But just because I'm not screaming or weeping, it doesn't mean I'm being strong: just emotionally shut down. In fact, I've been so weak that I haven't dared to feel.

The therapy gives me a deeper understanding of what has shaped me, and of the baggage I've been carrying. It has affected my capacity to process the shock of suddenly losing my child. My whole life has been marked by Mum's guilt games. I've already had emotional lockdowns before, and been so burdened by guilt that I didn't dare listen to my feelings. True, I could get angry like everyone else, but the anger was never visible on the outside. I didn't dare release it.

My parents imprinted on me that our family must look good. *We don't have any problems.* No wonder my mother blamed me and my husband for buying the car that John crashed in. Nor was it any surprise that she blamed John for making trouble for the family. In terms of our family pattern, of course, my son's death is an ugly blot on our copybook.

Calm in the soul

Everything's different now. I'm much stronger. I'm much more aware of my feelings. I stand up for who I am, let no one screw me over, object when people say stupid things. Now I call a halt when something doesn't feel right, both at work and with my mother. I set limits and say, *'No, I don't think so.'* These may seem baby steps, but for me they're huge strides forward.

I'm working on building up a completely different relationship with my daughter from the one Mum and I had. Now I venture to tell Amanda what it was like. Not needing to defend Mum any more feels good.

I used to be terribly touchy, and soaked up criticism like a sponge. I didn't know how to go about pleasing people. Now I've been given tools that help me relate to what people say. After ten therapy sessions, I'm at peace with myself and feel calm and in harmony. I'd never have dared hope for that.

Life is fragile. My own isn't like other mothers', but that's how it is. I've reached some kind of acceptance. If it hadn't been for John's car aquaplaning, if he'd never collided with that truck, something else might have happened. He might have been run over when he got off the bus.

I'm no longer angry because my son's dead. I don't rage against it any more. But I'm extremely disappointed that life didn't turn out as we'd hoped. I feel cheated out of the future and a life with John around. As for myself, I haven't the slightest fear of dying. Then I'll get to know what happens. There must be something more than just black nothingness. My hope is that I'll get to meet John there, on the other side.

Today, I no longer feel locked in the events bound up with the accident and our son's catastrophic death. I have a good life and can feel joy in what I have now, the near and dear people around me… And all the fine memories of John, too. My beloved son who will always be here in my heart, for the rest of my life.

CHAPTER 8

Threat system and other action systems

Nature has created us human beings to be highly fit for purpose. We have normal reactions to events that are actually unbearable for us, and that no one should have to experience. Unfortunately, however, grim disasters are the stuff of many people's everyday lives. People are constantly subjected to war, famine, natural disasters, abuse and dysfunctional families. The system that takes over in such situations is the defence action system, which is also commonly known as the fight-or-flight response.

Inside us, there are thus survival reactions and systems. But when the danger is over — and we are, in fact, safe without realising it — we may continue to behave as if we were still under threat. This creates problems for us and those who are close to us.

Flee, fight or play dead

When something frightens and threatens us humans to the degree that we feel our existence is in danger, we react at several levels. Trying to understand what we are experiencing, we look inside ourselves for past experiences that can help us act appropriately in the moment. We take action to survive.

The body interacts with the brain, which tries to find a suitable strategy. There are three options for survival: fleeing, fighting or 'lying down and playing dead' — that is, leaving the body mentally or dissociating.

Often, in the acute, perilous situation before we have 'decided', we momentarily 'freeze', as this state is commonly described. It has often been confused with 'lying down and playing dead'. When we freeze, we often become stock-still, take in every impression and try to determine which of the three strategies will maximise our chance of survival and minimise our suffering. This is no conscious choice, but an ultra-fast physical process.

Very many factors affect the outcome of the event and its future impact on us. Research shows that even certain levels of specific chemical substances in the brain during the traumatic situation affect whether we later suffer from post-traumatic stress disorder (PTSD).

Our inner systems

As noted in the previous chapter, all humans are biopsychosocial beings. Each individual includes several biological and emotional systems that are dominant on different occasions. These may be called 'action systems'. They are biopsychosocial, meaning that they involve biological, psychological and social factors, such as our age, genes, personality and family relationships.

Action systems are goal-oriented and affective. That is, they involve core needs and desires that organise feelings, perceptions, thoughts, memories and behaviours. Mammalian action systems include those that are concerned with attachment, caretaking, sociability, exploration, procreation, energy management, play and defence.

Trauma-generated imbalance

The attachment and sociability systems are dominant when we are safe, secure and in balance. Then, among others, the soothing attachment hormone oxytocin is released. The defence action system concerns our survival under threat.

Healthy people largely integrate their various needs, desires and associated action systems. However, in individuals with trauma-related dissociation, the diverse longings, strivings and the associated action systems are more disconnected and seldom work together. For example, they find it difficult to link and balance their attachment and other social needs and their defence interests. This said, conflicts among differing needs and desires are common. For example, healthy individuals may confuse their various needs, fail to grasp what they 'really' need or confuse the needs of human closeness and sexuality. However, they do not associate these conflicts and this lack of clarity with the development and maintenance of dissociative parts of their personality.

CHAPTER 9

Post-traumatic stress

In the first month after a traumatising event, we often suffer acute stress symptoms (acute stress disorder). These are normal reactions to a trying experience. At this stage, it is important for helpful people — if any — in the sufferers' vicinity to see what kind of reactions predominate. Those who have many dissociative symptoms should not, for example, be pushed or hurried into measures intended to give them insight. Sufferers need time, and sometimes quite a long time, before they can make progress towards the truth about what they have been through. During this time, they should not be pushed to visit places that make them anxious or undergo other experiences that arouse great fear and pain. Doing so may pose a risk of their recovery being more difficult and less complete.

Usually, we humans have very good healing ability. Most acute stress symptoms tend to heal by themselves relatively fast. But sometimes, the acute stress reaction gives way to post-traumatic stress disorder (PTSD). Instead of abating, the symptoms then become entrenched and grow over time. To be able to put the experience behind us, we need professional help.

If children undergo trauma of an isolated nature and receive help with their reactions, and are comforted and soothed, most children deal with this very well. But if children are exposed to physical and/or psychological trauma and then receive no help from adults in dealing with their reactions, the risk of traumatisation increases.

Secure enough to cope

We may suffer a simple form of PTSD after an event like a road accident, robbery, natural disaster or assault, or from witnessing a close relative being affected by a similar incident. We call these events traumatising: they *can* cause trauma wounds. After such an experience, we may have one or more unpleasant symptoms that persist for a long time. We may worry, be constantly tense, have trouble sleeping, have nightmares and start avoiding people, places or other things reminiscent of the experience. The memory of the event intrudes on us repeatedly. Anxiety, concentration difficulties and more disturb daily life.

Even if, in adulthood, we experience traumatic events that might inflict traumatic wounds on us, there is little risk of our suffering PTSD if we already have a secure foundation and are well cared for immediately after the trauma. If we repeatedly experience painful incidents in adulthood, our PTSD risk rises in line with their number, depending on such factors as the care we receive, our life situation and our fundamental security.

We react differently

How severely and adversely affected by trauma a person may be varies greatly. It is not the scale of the events they undergo that determines how traumatised people become. Whether trauma victims are considered to suffer from PTSD is a matter of their personal experience of what has happened and the extent of their symptoms.

These varying difficulties and symptoms can cause different degrees of suffering. For some people who have experienced terror and danger, PTSD may be the result. But others who have lived through the same kind of painful event and shown similar symptoms of acute stress may be symptom-free after a while, and never suffer from PTSD. Their symptoms have faded away.

It is not possible to predict exactly which individuals will incur post-traumatic stress. Researchers have shown that hormone concentrations immediately after the trauma can provide clues. Measuring stress hormones can offer relatively good insight into what the effects will be. But it does not give the whole truth. In addition, it is hardly possible to measure hormone levels in everyone who undergoes painful events, and thereby identify who needs treatment.

What causes traumatisation also depends on many different factors. We are affected by when in life the trauma occurs, our early attachment pattern, our vulnerability, whether we have undergone repeated traumatic experiences and the care and recognition we received when they occurred.

It happened to me

When a traumatic event has affected someone, it must be gradually integrated into the person's entire consciousness. *This did happen to me, but it happened then, not now.* Integration needs to take place at every level in the victim: in thoughts, emotions and body alike. Being subjected to extreme stress often means that our capacity to integrate the experience decreases.

Examples of factors that can be protective and boost our integrative capacity are a well-developed, secure attachment pattern, good relationships and the experience of recovering from previous difficulties. Reaching the age of 25 before being affected by trauma seems to improve this ability.

The PTSD diagnosis

Post-traumatic stress affects the whole person. Our body and our mental state are inseparable. Structural, chemical and electrical changes take place in the brain. The body stores memories and constantly reacts as if we are under threat.

The PTSD diagnosis is characterised by four symptom categories. The diagnosis is made only if these symptoms are present and at least a month has passed since the event. To meet the diagnostic criteria, people must have either experienced at least one external event that involved being affected by or witnessing death or a threat of death, a severe injury or sexual violence, or learnt that someone close to them have been affected by such events.

The four symptom categories are:

- Hyperarousal (feeling 'on edge')
- Re-experiencing
- Avoidance
- Negative changes.
- These four categories vary in extent from one person to another.

Many different symptoms

Hyperarousal includes such symptoms as insomnia, angry outbursts, irritability, concentration difficulties, excessive watchfulness and being easily startled.

Re-experiencing involves recurrent, intrusive recollections of the event, nightmares, flashbacks, physical reactions and sensitivity to the kind of stimulus that can trigger the re-experiencing. All the memories may persist as incoherent fragments in the form of odours, sounds, tastes, feelings and images that are associated with the event and bring back unpleasant memories.

The third symptom category is *avoidance*, which means a constant attempt to avoid experiencing stimuli associated with the trauma. These may be feelings, thoughts or a scent, taste or sound that causes an all-pervasive unpleasant feeling. This may mean that sufferers start avoiding people, places and other things reminiscent of the event. Other effects may be memory loss and reduced interest in what we used to enjoy. We may feel shut down, as if inside a bubble. We are observers, without feelings. It may be difficult to look ahead. We live in both the 'trauma time' and the present. Putting events behind ourselves is difficult. The more severely traumatised we are, the more our sense of time is confused.

Negative changes are a matter of incurring difficulties, in thoughts and mood, with memory, feelings of guilt and shame, and despondency and depression.

If we have had a reasonably secure life and sound self-esteem before the event occurred, these facilitate our return to normal. Our PTSD is then usually easy to treat and is often called simple PTSD. More severe forms are known as complex PTSD. Today, 'complex PTSD' is a term widely used by professionals and included in one of the two biggest diagnostic manuals as a diagnosis in its own right.

Triggers

Thus, hidden, threatening and overwhelming feelings do not die. They are encapsulated deep inside us where they smoulder, unseen. Suddenly they flare up, setting off apparently strange emotional reactions in our everyday lives. How does this happen?

We humans constantly connect what we are experiencing here and now with our memories of past experiences. Without being aware of it, we associate new impressions with what we have known and experienced before in our lives. Accordingly, our memories live on as disconnected fragments in the form of scents, sounds, tastes, feelings and images associated with past events. A trigger is something that activates these stored fragments.

Triggers can come from outside — perhaps the smell of sweat and stale beer, a visual impression like a stranger's posture in the street, or an anxiety-generating location. A trigger can also come from within: it may be a thought, a physical sensation or a feeling.

If our past experiences are associated with negative feelings, triggers can arouse anxiety, worry, anger and other strong feelings. They alert us to imminent danger. They set off an alarm inside us, at top volume: *Warning! There may be a threat nearby.*

Insecurity's icy grip

Important factors that affect people's degree of personal vulnerability during a traumatic event include how early on the experiences of trauma take place and, in general, the care provided for them. Had they previously, as children, had a chance to learn how to regulate their feelings? Are there, or have there been, people close by who offer, or have offered, means of repairing the harm done to them?

Repeated traumatising events can make a person's condition worse. This makes the question of whether the individual has managed to develop a basically secure attachment pattern even more important. If not, the risk of severe traumatisation is greater.

Did the traumatising experiences begin at an early age? Was it an attachment person who subjected the child to them, and were the experiences repeated, perhaps taking place regularly? If so, the vulnerability is immense. Attachment patterns are frequently disorganised and, if so, lengthen the road to symptom-free, stable everyday life.

Varying degrees of traumatisation and dissociation are explored below. It is enormously important to take the state a person is in with the utmost seriousness. One must listen carefully to find out: *How severely traumatised is this person? What would help this particular individual?*

Let us now trace Oscar's path from his childhood traumas to a more balanced adult life. We take up his story just before he reaches the finishing line as a winner over his past, fully integrated and stable.

THIRD STORY

Until the age of 39, Oscar tries to live as normal a life as possible. He has toiled and struggled to get his life on track. After completing his education, he has gone in for a career, got married and had children. His efforts have been shaped by numerous wishes about what his life should contain. Oscar has created a great deal, but he is far from happy.

Overwhelming experiences in his early life have brought serious consequences. Fighting to build a functioning life on a severely damaged foundation calls for a great abundance of energy. It wears him down, mentally and physically. For Oscar, headaches, stomach pain and anxiety are constant companions. Relationships suffer and he feels as if he is not truly participating in life. Eventually, he comes extremely close to a burnout. Then he takes the decision to go into therapy.

Twelve years and three therapists later, Oscar steps into TT's reception. He brings his latest therapist, whose own supervisor has provided the contact. The therapist and supervisor have been concerned about what can help Oscar, and with genuine thoughtfulness conclude that he needs more specific trauma treatment. Oscar agrees to the suggestion.

He knows there are several parts of himself, but does not really understand how everything is connected. How is he to succeed in moving on?

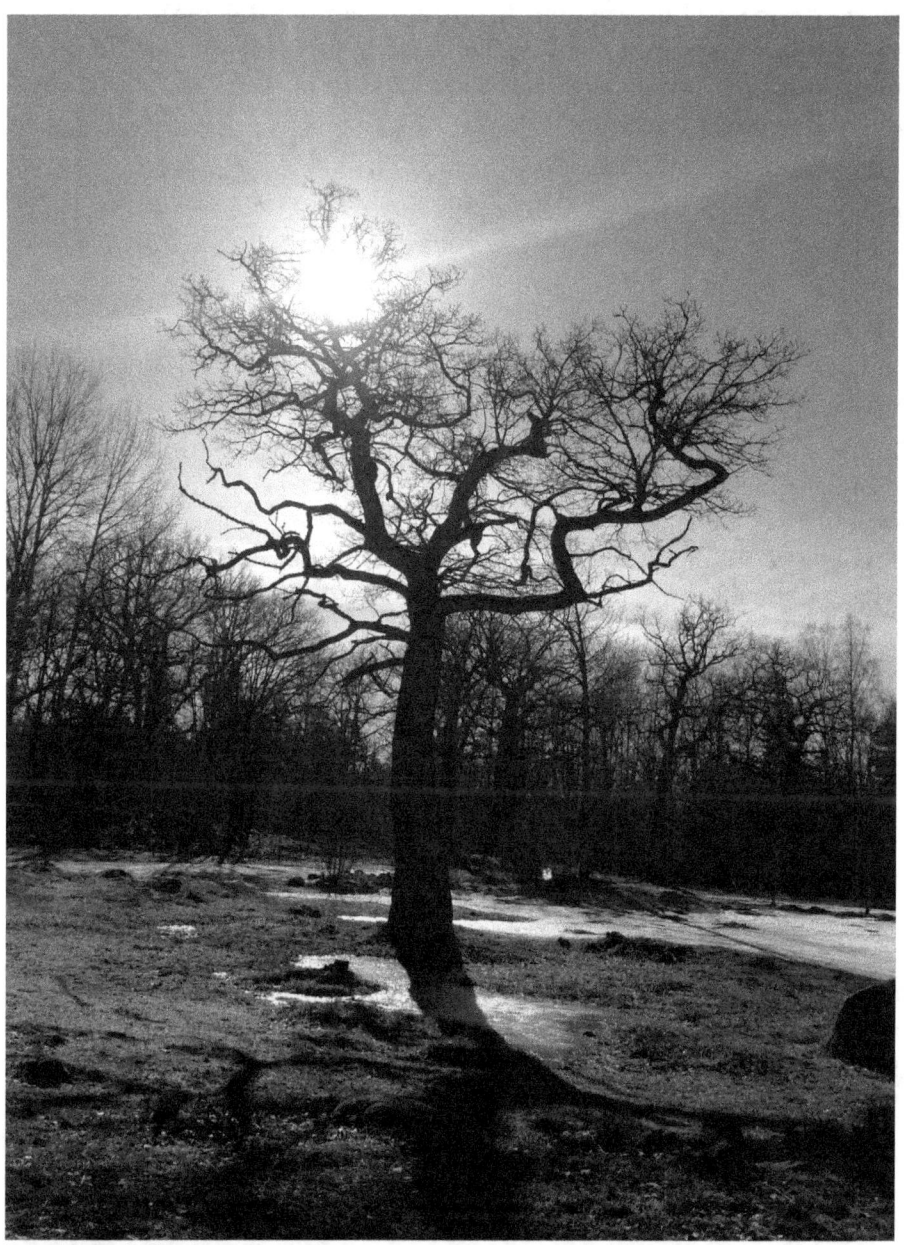

By Annica Lilja Ljung

Oscar

Oscar grew up in an apparently ordinary family. Below the surface, something was terribly wrong. To survive, he disconnected all the unpleasant memories and feelings, and shut in the scared little boy and the angry, powerful youth.

'That's how I survived — by distancing myself from everything that overwhelmed me with terror. Now, the parts of my personality are merging together more and more. We share the present and everything we've been through. Becoming integrated like this is infinitely pleasant.'

For a long time, I tried to live in the conviction that I had a completely ordinary childhood. At the same time, I felt something was very seriously wrong.

I isolated and limited myself. As soon as a relationship became too close, it all felt extremely difficult. That applied to both friends and girls. I switched off, fooling myself into believing I had a great need to be alone. I sort of tried to 'think myself into' being normal. But I didn't understand what a normal life means.

Now I'm sad to have missed so much. I've been terribly closed-in, unable to find out about life.

Dark cloud

I grew up in a middle-class family with Mum, Dad and two elder brothers. Everything new was extremely difficult for me, every change hard to cope with. When I left upper secondary school in my home town, Borlänge, I moved to Stockholm to study at the Royal Institute of Technology. Living alone in a new place felt awful, and going to the Institute filled me with anxiety. Stockholm became like a big dark cloud over me. In the end, I was forced to stop studying for a semester. Getting there simply became too difficult.

I had a girlfriend, but the relationship ended. Somehow, I managed to complete my studies, and moved home to Borlänge to take up my first job as an engineer. In due course I met Eva, my wife-to-be. Together, we moved to Stockholm, where the career opportunities were.

We got married and had children. I worked a tremendous lot and got horribly close to having a burnout. Paternity leave was my salvation.

Small and vulnerable

But I still didn't feel well. I was plagued by ailments, such as more or less constant tension headaches and stomach pains. One day, a mother at our son's nursery said she was in therapy after burnout and sexual abuse. That got me thinking about whether I should go into therapy. Might it improve my poor mental state? Somewhere inside, I knew that I'd been abused too. Quite soon, I contacted Matt, the hypnotherapist that the mother at the nursery was seeing.

Trying hypnosis was a powerful experience. Even in the first session, I went into a trance. Everything became increasingly clear. Masses of images came to me. At first, it was more a matter of symbolic pictures, but eventually it became more real. It was like watching a film.

This is how I remember the first symbolic images. I see the garden at my grandfather's house. Small and alone, I lie in the hammock under the big trees, looking towards the food cellar. Then Dad comes. He climbs out of the basement and into the garden. Dad walks up to me with his trousers unbuttoned. He has an erection.

His erect penis, with its pointed tip, shines like a light bulb. The situation is very threatening. I know his sexual organ has harmed me and will hurt me again.

Up to the surface

Under hypnosis, I usually never experienced any feelings at all. It was like looking through a camera lens. I viewed myself from outside, with no emotional overlay. Very often, I didn't dare go into my body and sense the vileness there.

As the sessions with the hypnotherapist went by, the picture of my childhood became clearer. Memories that part of me had lacked access to, but that I realise I've borne inside me all my life, rose to the surface. At the same time, I had to relive the traumatic events over and over again. As the therapy progressed, too, recollections from a very early age crystallised. I was a very young boy, with no language, full of incomprehensible feelings. Even when I was in the pram, Dad was the big storm cloud in my world. The fear was overwhelming.

But I've lived such a 'normal' life with career, wife and children, I've never broken down or had to be put in a psychiatric clinic — could all this really have happened to me? My thoughts gave me no peace of mind. In the end, I decided to confront my family. My middle brother Simon was the first person I contacted.

Liberating affirmation

When I told Simon about my suspicions, he replied plainly: *'When you said you wanted to talk about something important, I knew this was what you were going to say.'* Getting affirmation right away felt really good. Simon said he thought he'd also been sexually abused by our father, but that he didn't want to delve into the past.

It felt enormously liberating that my brother said he was abused too. Now I wasn't alone any more. His answer gave me the strength to confront our parents.

Dad's response came quickly: *'I have no memory of it.'* Mum's reply was the same. When I turned to my eldest brother Peter, I got the same message: *'I don't remember anything about that.'*

Instead of giving up, I went on asking questions about events in our childhood.

Truth creeps out

Memories of the abuse continued to plague me. Over a long period, I went to Dad's home maybe once a week, hoping for confirmation of what had happened. Now and again, I was angry and threatening. At other times, I rubbed him up the right way, promised not to criticise him and begged him to tell me, because the truth would help me. I also arranged meetings with my whole family to try to get confessions and more information about what had happened.

These bizarre family gatherings went on for quite a while. Dad shielded himself from the truth. No doubt he wasn't up to admitting what he'd done. Mum went on being evasive, but it gradually emerged how worried she'd been when Dad was at home. During the week, when he'd worked in another town, it was nice and quiet at our place, she said. But at weekends and during holidays when Dad was at home and Mum had gone to bed, she'd sometimes heard one of us boys crying. *Why didn't she get up and console us, then? Why didn't she find out why we were upset?*

Later on, my mother confirmed that she had been present during the assaults I'd confronted her about.

Helpless victim

The hypnotherapy continued weekly for almost six years. Mental pictures of sexual abuse welled up. Facing incidents I'd carried inside me for so long did me good. I'd really known all the time, but now what I'd been through became clear.

But I felt I was stuck in identifying myself as a powerless victim. Matt, the therapist, said, *'I understand that you can never forgive this.'* That irreconcilable stance was his only image of what was possible. The therapy gave me no tools for getting away from that self-image, so making progress was difficult. Finally, Matt thought my treatment was complete. There I stood, under the leaden weight of memories, filled with implacable anger. What was I to do with all these 'new' memories? I had no idea how to move on.

Several parts of me

Another therapist, Lena, was recommended to me by friends. She had a different approach: she realised that I'd had to relive the abuse during the hypnotherapy, without being helped to work through my trauma. She saw how I was stuck with that bag of painful memories. I felt hate, but that hate wasn't me.

Somehow, Lena conveyed her feeling that *it's appalling, what you've been through.* That fuelled my self-image as a victim. But one important step forward was that she saw and understood that there were several parts of me. Unfortunately, I didn't feel she could help me get in touch with all these parts. After two years' therapy, I realised that my hatred was an obstacle to me. I'd resumed contact with my brothers and mother. Now I realised they too were victims, not perpetrators — and that gave me access to my love both for myself and for them. By then, I felt I'd reached the end of the road with that therapist. I needed to move on.

Everyone can join in

My third therapist, Ingrid, realised I had some type of PTSD that I needed help in getting over. Unlike her predecessors, she was aware of her own limitations and realised I needed trauma-focused therapy. I'm immensely grateful that Ingrid helped me find my way to TT.

With TT, everything was different. I and the dissociative parts of my personality met clear respect and interest. In previous therapy, not all my parts had been able to appear with the same clarity. TT talked in a special way — with complete openness, as if to all of us — right from the start. She was keen for us to feel welcome. It was so considerate and reassuring.

I'd already grasped that I had different parts of me, but I wasn't aware of how they were actually interconnected, or who they were. TT understood clearly that the adult Oscar wasn't the only one sitting there in the room. She wanted to meet every single one of my parts. All were welcome and joined in.

Locked-in feelings

There were hundreds of children of different ages in me — from toddlers to teens. It was a tough job, but while I was seeing TT they successively merged into three dominant parts of my personality: the little guy, the powerful one and the adult Oscar.

My survival strategy has been to largely turn off my feelings. All these years, my adult, competent everyday self has been dominant. My feelings have been locked inside the little guy and the powerful one, keeping the painful stuff away so that the adult part of me can function in daily life. That insight has come quite late, but now I see it clearly.

I want all three parts to be heard here in the book. In the past, we were unaware of one another. The mutual discovery terrified us, but over time we've become increasingly united.

The little guy's story

For a long time, I lived as if in the dark. I was so scared and unable to take part in life here and now. In the therapy with Matt and Lena, I hid to prevent them from seeing me. I wasn't sure they'd treat me in a way that felt safe; I had to try and protect myself. That's why I became invisible. I liked Lena — she was loving, and I'd been missing that all my life. Still, I didn't dare step forth and talk to her.

At first, I was afraid of TT as well. I didn't know who she was. Soon I saw she herself had no fear. That was wonderful, and made me a little less scared.

After a while, I ventured forth more and more. TT was kind and offered protection. I had to imagine us building a fence around me, to guard against the powerful one who frightened me so much. He reminded me so much of Dad. Inside the protective fence, I became calmer. The powerful one got to build a house for himself, where he could feel safe. Then I understood he'd been as scared as I had. We needed our protected zones.

The children dare to emerge

With TT's support, we created a beautiful meadow to be in, with Swedish ginger snaps and strawberry cordial on offer. Children came from every direction. They'd been hiding in the woods, but now ventured into the lovely, safe, protected meadow. They sat around in a circle and ate the biscuits. A girl started telling everyone what had happened: that her father had forced himself on her and she'd transformed herself from a boy into a girl to get away. The other children sat around listening, without challenging or judging her.

More and more of them wanted to talk about what they'd been through. Three boys had undergone the same experience: each one's father had driven his penis down the boy's throat so he couldn't breathe. They were all relieved by being allowed to tell their stories. When the children had finished their own stories, it was as if they dissolved and became part of me. We shared an ever expanding portion of reality.

Suddenly, one day, the powerful one ran out of his house, came out to us in the meadow and sat down some distance away from me. Everyone stayed sitting there. In some strange way, we'd come so far now that we were no longer afraid of him. I saw that he was a child, just like the rest of us. After a while, he began telling his story.

The powerful one speaks

For a long time (he said), I'd got on fine standing there alone in my house, looking out. I'd seen how good the children felt about relating their experiences. I was so ashamed of my own past — of having been like Dad. Running out to the others in the meadow and putting what had happened into words was a huge relief. It made me realise those terrible days were over — that vileness was no longer happening.

The sessions with TT made my days easier. The nights were still harrowing, with many nightmares. Then, it was more difficult to remember that the abuse belongs forever in the past. After each therapy session, we tried to summarise our experiences. The parts of my personality began to interact more and more, outside the treatment room too. Finally, only the three of us were left.

I've always been terrified of the little guy's strong feelings. As for him, the power in me has petrified him. The adult part has distanced itself from us both, trying to fend off our emotional sides. He too, in fact, was very scared. The fear is still with us, but we talk more and more concretely and are starting to understand one another better.

The adult one speaks

Nowadays, we three have progressed enough to share what we've been through. We can all tell our stories, but maybe it's a bit easier for me. After all, I'm used to staying in my thoughts and putting feelings aside.

The therapy created opportunities to process the grim events of my childhood — to let go of, and deal with, all the repressed feelings. Even as a very young child, I was subjected to sexual molestation.

One early memory is from the age of three. I'm lying naked on my parents' bed, and Dad is assaulting me. Mum comes into the bedroom and holds my hands down. Inside me, the pain is severe.

Much later, Mum and I talked about it and she confirmed Dad's abuse. But she played down what happened, excusing it: in her version, Dad had 'just' masturbated over me — and she didn't pin down my hands, just held them to console me. But in my world, the pain was overwhelming and Mum did nothing to stop him. Even when I was so young that I was still sleeping in a cot in their bedroom, Dad used me on several occasions to succeed in having sex with Mum. He fingered my penis to get excited, so that he could have sex with her.

Mum's betrayal

Over time, I became more and more involved in my parents' intercourse. Maybe Dad chose to get Mum involved in his acts to prevent her from gossiping…? She too enjoyed using me, I remember.

Dad orders me to lick Mum's genitalia. She gets aroused. Dad masturbates and gets very turned on by watching. I'm about six or seven years old. The whole business feels incomprehensible and wrong. Both Dad and Mum seem threatening, so I protect myself by kind of switching off. Part of me dies.

It was like living in two different realities. In the daytime, the apparently ordinary family life went on. For Mum, what the façade looked like — keeping up appearances — was what mattered most. In the evening and at night, things were totally different. No limits. Threatening. Home was no safe place. For me, there was no connection between these two realities. The terror sometimes seeped through into everyday life, but I switched it off as best I could.

Desire to punish

Being able, during the therapy, to safely bring out all the dark, remembered images, still and moving, has really helped. The fact that every part of me dared to come forward and put his experiences into words was crucial for understanding and integrating what I'd been through. The questioning thoughts can still appear at times: *What if that never happened? What if it's not true?*

But I realise not all such thoughts are relevant. I know that what happened really did happen, and that it went on for a very long time. What's more, I've had parts of the events confirmed by my mother, although she distanced herself from the events and played them down.

How could Dad and Mum do this to me? Perhaps I'll never understand why my parents acted as they did, but I've accepted that my upbringing was like that.

The assaults became ever more frequent and aggravated. I remember how I lay on the bed, like a corpse, with Dad on top. Recall how he sat on top of me, with his bottom on my face. His anus was suffocating me: I couldn't get air. Apparently, it was titillating for Dad to govern me, to control whether I'd live or die.

Dad's sexual pleasure and lust to punish me went hand in hand. The assaults now took place not only at night. They could just as easily happen in the daytime, in the boiler room down in the basement.

Dad's friend

I'm convinced that Dad had a very marked preference for children and men, rather than women. He travelled a lot and made new male friends. One year, he wasn't even planning to come home for Christmas. He'd met a man called Hans and wanted to be with him. Then Mum said: *'Can't he come along? Bring Hans, and come home to celebrate Christmas.'* So that's what happened.

I firmly believe that Dad tempted Hans by the fact that there were children there at home. It turned out I was expected to be present when they had sex. At first, I had to fondle their penises. Then they took turns shoving their erect penises into my mouth. When Dad or Hans pushed their genitals down into my throat and ejaculated, it felt like I would choke.

Dad's friend lived with us for six months. Our whole family life was strained. Mum was very weak, letting the abuse happen again and again.

Relief and shame

My middle brother Simon suffered from Dad's lack of limits too. Simon was far from well mentally, as his obsessive-compulsive behaviour and strange rituals showed. A fork lying at slightly the wrong angle on the dining table could set off a meltdown — he'd yell and scream, and couldn't eat for several hours. That frightened me.

We boys had been given our own rooms. In the dark, late at night, I lay listening through the thin wall between Simon's room and mine. Would Dad come into mine or go into his? If he went into Simon's room, I could exhale. *What a relief!* But when I heard Simon's desperate sobbing, I was ashamed. I thought he'd go crazy.

I was just a little boy lying there alone in the dark, terrified that my beloved brother would die. And I thought: *If I don't resist next time, will they come back to me instead, and leave Simon in peace, maybe?*

Paedophile visitors

Dad continued coming to my room at night and, as time went on, the violence increased. Controlling and dominating me were tremendously exciting for Dad. For instance, he used a battery that he connected to my genitals to give me electric shocks. It hurt terribly.

Sometimes Dad brought friends home. Hans was just the first: more followed. Charlie was one of them.

On one occasion, in the middle of the day, Dad and Charlie tied me to the carpentry bench down in the basement. Then they raped me anally. It was like Dad treated Charlie to it — to using me. Afterwards, I was supposed to pull up my trousers and leave as if nothing had happened. Mum was at home. She must have understood that something wasn't right.

Victims and perpetrators

At some point, Dad began to involve us children in committing the abuse. To start with, he got my eldest brother Peter involved in the assaults. Dad stood next to us and masturbated while he gave my big brother orders.

For me, it felt very threatening that there were two of them. I had no one to ally myself with, either physically or mentally. If Dad thought I needed an extra smack on the nose, the abuse immediately became even more brutal.

At a later stage, Dad forced me to take part in the assaults on Peter. It was terrible to have to abuse my brother. I felt that I was completely in my Dad's power, and thinking about that makes me feel awful.

Looking back, I've understood that Dad was increasing his power even more in this way. By turning both Mum and us, the children, into perpetrators he was able to rule and control the whole family.

Frightened into silence

The family was an ocean of insecurity. From infancy until my early teens, I was exposed to numerous assaults. The rapes got worse and worse. I perceived that Dad got pleasure when I felt I was choking. He must have sensed my panic and known I wouldn't dare bite him in an effort to defend myself.

Only once did I try to tell someone about the abuse. My maternal grandmother and grandfather lived on a farm in the countryside. I told Gran that Dad wasn't kind to me. Then she went to Dad and asked what that was about. The result was that he punished me by almost suffocating me. After that, I never said anything else. Instead, I kept a low profile. Made myself invisible.

For a long time, I thought I'd die if I snitched. Even today, it feels like I'm being disobedient, sitting here and telling you about it. On my way here to the interview, I was overcome by anxiety. It felt like I had Dad's penis in my throat, preventing me from speaking.

Switched off

When I was 13, I couldn't take it any more. One night, half deliberately and half by mistake, I pushed Dad out of bed. After that he tried to return once more, but then never again.

Still, the abuse has continued to shape my existence — my teenage and adult life, studies and career, parenthood and relationships. My trauma has made me extremely inaccessible when it comes to the romantic and sexual sides of life. While I've wanted intimacy, I've been afraid to reveal myself. I've had a kind of shell to protect myself and it's spoilt my relationships. Although I've longed for closeness, I've been so scared of becoming defenceless if I didn't have that emotional shelter. So I withdrew, stayed on my own and understood nothing.

Moment of truth

For long periods, I've had no contact at all with my family of origin. When Dad was dying, I went to the hospital, hoping to finally get a confession. Both Dad and I realised he didn't have much time left. I asked him to give me confirmation that the abuse had really happened.

I began by asking if he'd molested my big brother Peter. Dad nodded. Then I asked whether he'd abused me too. Another nod. When I inquired whether he'd also assaulted my middle brother, no answer came. Dad closed his eyes and withdrew into himself. He couldn't bring himself to admit abusing Simon.

No one could imagine

I've brooded a lot. *Why didn't I become an alcoholic? A prescription-drug addict? Or a junkie?* That would have helped me escape from all the horrible memories. *Why haven't I been locked up in a psychiatric clinic? Killed myself?*

Maybe it was my salvation that part of my childhood was nonetheless apparently 'normal'. I mean… we weren't destitute. We had food on the table. Clean clothes. I went to school. No one had a clue what was going on behind closed doors.

Longing for love

My middle brother Simon suffered greatly. I think that led to a decline in the assaults on him. My big brother Peter fled from home as soon as he could. In middle school, he was already spending the weekends with our maternal grandparents in the countryside. I think that was his way of escaping the abuse.

I, the youngest, was the only one left and felt that the abuse was happening increasingly often. At the same time, Dad got a taste for ever more perverted acts, and I felt terribly vulnerable and alone. I feel bitter about that. In my fantasies, I was utterly convinced that Dad and Mum would kill me if I told anyone what was going on at our home. I perceived that they were both extremely afraid of it getting out.

Inside me, there was a silent longing for Mum and Dad to love me, to give me affectionate hugs. But the only purpose of my existence was to satisfy their needs. And I felt really bad, as if it was my fault. Mrs Karlsson, our cleaning lady, was the only one who ever gave me a kind hug.

Darkness over me

When I'd confronted my family, I decided to contact Dad's old friend Tom. He seemed to be a good, kind person. Tom told me he'd suspected early on that Dad had molested us boys. When my brother Simon had developed obsessive thoughts, Dad asked Tom to help him find a child psychologist, but at a place other than home in Borlänge. Everything was to be done discreetly.

I got more pieces of the puzzle from Tom. He knew that Dad had tried, several times, to pick up younger guys in the saunas at clubs they'd visited together. Once, Tom had asked Dad bluntly whether he was abusing us children at home. The answer had been extremely unclear and evasive.

Tom said he'd been worried about me, and seen sadness in my eyes, even when I laughed. He saw a dark shadow hanging over me. But he never intervened.

Seeing the truth

Ordinary sex didn't suffice to satisfy my father. His thirst for power grew, and the assaults got rougher and more aggressive. Sometimes I wonder why Dad turned out as he did. His mother died when he was a little boy. He grew up with his father and his deeply religious aunt in a world of lies, full of double standards.

Perhaps Dad felt a powerful urge to challenge the limits of morality? Maybe strong sexual expression was his way of trying to suppress anxiety? I don't know. But I know he hurt me very deeply indeed.

For me, it's important to see things as they really are, and not have any illusions. I've tried to get to the bottom of things, and left no stone unturned. That's my driving force: seeing the truth, and daring to face what comes to light.

Never again do I want to live a lie. I'm making sure the family secrets don't roll over to the next generation. So it feels important to tell my story without protecting anyone.

All together

The trauma therapy with TT has revolutionised my life. Before, I had to completely disconnect important parts of me, forgetting both the little guy and the powerful one in me. After all, that's how I've survived: by distancing myself from all the feelings that overwhelmed me with the utmost terror — all so that the everyday adult person would have the strength to get through daily life.

In the therapy, I got in touch with parts inside me that I hadn't known about, but that had affected me to the max. When I saw what important work the little guy and the powerful one were doing out in the meadow with all the other children, I felt: *Now at last something can happen!* I saw that it was good for them to tell their life stories. That became an important turning point. For the first time, I felt real hope. Instead of controlling and avoiding difficult situations in my life, I was able to face the disquiet felt by the little guy and the powerful one. It was like getting a toolbox that I could start using to move on. It was almost magical.

The adult Oscar speaks

I, the adult, was able talk to these parts of my personality and make them realise that the abuse is no longer happening and that we no longer live in the childhood home with my parents. The little guy and the powerful one were disoriented in time and space. Now they could understand better where they were, and in which period, and it enabled them to see the world with different eyes.

They realised that all they knew was memories of the time when the assaults were taking place. Now, on the other hand, there was nothing to be afraid of and, what was more, there was me — the adult. The more I can share feelings and thoughts with the powerful one and the little guy, the more we're integrated into a single person and the less we're governed by childhood feelings and memories.

Now I dare let out every part of me. I don't want to keep a distance from the others any more. It feels great to hear the powerful one and the little guy when they step forward. It feels very good when we're all gathered together.

The powerful one speaks

For very many years, I made myself invisible. The little guy and I were hiding, both from each other and from the therapists. I was very much alone. The years of hypnotherapy were hard going for me.

Twice a week, we went there and re-experienced the terror and vulnerability. That took diabolical strength. It was very hard to relive everything. The abuse was repeated. Then I had to protect myself and hide even more. Sometimes I became manic. At home, I fixed and renovated things at a furious pace.

My own perception of being powerful has been complicated. Dad was strong too, and cast a huge dark shadow. That negative force is scary.

Now, in retrospect, I think the time in hypnotherapy reliving the trauma filled me with great bitterness towards my family. I couldn't see clearly that Dad was the perpetrator and the others were victims. Reliving it meant that I filled up with hatred. I cleared away a lot in my life, because I was convinced that all the problems were outside me. It hurts to think about how I acted, in a way I now regret.

The powerful one says more

When we came to TT, I realised that here was a person I could neither fool nor hide from. I felt truly welcome. It was good, but hard work at first. Telling my story was a huge relief. Then I became less lonely. But I really felt I was taking a big risk. Telling the story was perilous. I lived with the conviction that I'd actually be killed if I revealed the family secrets.

TT succeeded in making me secure enough to dare. For a long time, I stood there alone in my house, watching the children in the meadow. Kids of all ages came there, from the youngest, who could barely walk to teenage boys, nearly grown up. One after another, they came forward and told their stories. No one was punished. It was a great relief when I finally dared to run out of my protective home, step into the circle and tell my story.

More key words from the powerful one

To some extent, I'm still scared and angry about what happened. It wasn't okay! It enrages me that Mum didn't take us away from there. She was a cowardly wretch who failed in her duty as a mother.

But now I'm no longer alone. I step forward without that uncontrolled, scary force. I never take over and do things the adult Oscar is unaware of. Before, when I barged in and took command, he couldn't remember what had happened.

We bear our wounds together — the little guy, the adult Oscar and I. We share our past and have learnt the benefits of forgiveness. I was terrified at first when, a bit hesitantly, we started socialising with the family. It's been a great boon getting new perspectives, and seeing that we were all victims, apart from Dad. Before, I was terribly angry with my big brother Peter. Speeding up forgiveness is hard. But finally we were able to meet.

The little guy's present day

I've been desperately afraid all my life. Of Dad and Mum, of my big brother, of all the dangerous men who Dad brought home — everything and everyone, really. I was scared stiff of being killed.

The turning point came with TT. But it took a long time. Previously, I'd had no conscious contact with the powerful one. The more he showed himself, the more afraid I became. When he became manic, he seemed as threatening as Dad. Terrified, I ran and hid. It really helped that, in the therapy, TT supported me in creating a zone protected by a fence around me. For me, it was a great relief when the powerful one stayed inside his house for long periods and focused his power on something other than me. I used to be afraid of him; now, I no longer need to be. There's no danger now. We've broken the mould.

In the past, I've been unable to participate in this life. I couldn't understand it, and was incapable of living here and now. For a long time, I thought I was still living with Dad and Mum in Borlänge. With TT's help, I managed to move to Stockholm. At night, it was as if I moved back to that dangerous life in Borlänge, but after a while I was able to grasp the fact that I'm living in safety here in Stockholm.

The adult Oscar tells more

In the past, I was more shut in. That doesn't happen so often now. I'm aware of which of the different parts of me is talking and acting. It's a tremendously good feeling, daring to let the emotional and vulnerable parts of me step forward. Now we're more in unison. Feelings and actions belong together.

I now understand how I locked my feelings inside, in the little guy and the powerful one. That created resistance and drained my energy. How did we get past all the obstacles? By talking to one another. Listening. In the therapy, we learnt physical exercises that helped us bond. Our highly charged emotional experiences were expressed in my hands, which we used to symbolise us, the various parts of our personality. We genuinely felt we were located in the two hands, the little guy in one hand and the powerful one in the other. Step by step we were able to achieve closeness with one another simply through sheer physical movements, and to feel how close we could get.

Now that we've become more and more welded together, I feel that all the parts are involved in everyday life. For example, if I have an important meeting to attend at work, I check what the powerful one and the little guy are feeling and thinking. I listen and then say, *'You don't have to act. I'll take responsibility for this.'* They're at the meeting too, but make no contribution. Before, I used to cut off those parts of me and wasn't completely there. Now I can be strong and come forward in a better way.

The adult Oscar on life today

I feel much freer now, in touch with my feelings and my potential. I venture to say what I think and feel neither inferior nor subservient. At work, I'm more proactive and can use the powerful one's energy constructively. My colleagues find me more accessible and honest.

As I see it, I find myself at a stage of life where I'm testing my limits. I see my limitations, dare to challenge them and notice my own reaction when I overcome them. I understand how much I've let my trauma hold me back and rule my life. I used to see myself as a passive victim. I didn't think I could do anything about the terror and anxiety I carried inside. The sense of powerlessness generated even more worries and fears.

I used to be unable to see what had caused my limitations. Instead, I blamed external circumstances that had hit me. Facing what I've been through and understanding how it shaped me have been crucial. You might say I've had to re-evaluate others and myself alike.

More from the adult Oscar

Before, I believed it was my role to help and serve others. It was like a kind of addiction — I hardly knew how to relax otherwise. I didn't feel I deserved a good life. Nowadays, I seek people who don't lay all their problems in my lap. I choose positive relationships.

Unfortunately, both my professional and my family life have been governed by my limitations. I've rejected a good many job offers. Terrified of failing, I've made myself an underdog and not dared to stand out or believe in my capacity. I've never ventured to go all out for anything.

My marriage also suffered. My relationship with my then wife Eva was rigidly ruled by what I could cope with. Several years ago, when I got a chance to work abroad, we decided to move there. It was a big adjustment for the whole family, of course. I found changes terribly difficult, but I hoped that, if I lived far away from Sweden, I'd no longer be identified with my past.

Leaving Sweden

Unfortunately, moving abroad was a terrifying ordeal for me. My old trauma went into overdrive. It felt like all the awfulness was happening in the present. Instead of my getting away from it all, everything got worse.

When the boss demanded something from me, it felt like he was a perpetrator. My trauma was brought to bear on the present day. Time and space were mixed up, and at night I was tormented by horrible nightmares.

When I was in an office meeting there, in the big foreign city, if police sirens were suddenly audible it was enough to set me off. Panic-stricken, part of me was convinced my parents were coming to collect me and hurt me. *'Who do you think you are?'* came their shout. It was all happening inside my head, of course, but for me it was real.

I lasted two months. Then we all travelled home. My fear of failure made me fail.

Integrated and whole

I want to tell my story to show what a complete change has taken place. Today, I feel I have a considerably better rapport with my ex-wife. We have a more adult relationship now than when we were married. She no longer meets a terrified little boy in me.

I get on better with my kids, too. In the past, I didn't dare release them from my control. I felt I had to protect them in every way. Now they're in their teens and I can handle the fact that they're liberating themselves. It's healthy and good.

Today, what's happening around me no longer feels so important. I can take setbacks and challenges. I don't react with anxiety and fear anything like as strongly as I did. That makes life easier to live.

The parts of my personality are merging more and more. Before, we weren't even aware of one another. The mutual discovery scared us stiff. Now, we're joining in the same context. Sometimes it feels like we're talking simultaneously, with a common voice, and all three of us feel the same thing. Together, we breathe deeply and enjoy ourselves. Becoming integrated like this is really, really wonderful.

We're a unit. That gives me courage and strength.

CHAPTER 10

Degrees of traumatisation

All those who are traumatised are somewhere along the trauma scale, with more or fewer symptoms. Their traumatisation varies in complexity and has differing individual consequences. To be able to provide the right treatment, it is crucial to grasp *how* traumatised a person is.

Treatment methods based on an approach that includes neither similarities nor differences between simple and complex PTSD tend to be inadequate in helping the survivor of complex traumatisation all the way to achieving a balanced life. Neither can methods that disregard dissociative syndromes create proper healing.

Many therapists and methods focus on starting with the thin end of the wedge, modifying patients' thinking to enable them to see, in the moment, something that helps them realise that past horrors are over and done with. These are good and vital but insufficient perceptions. Seeing the bigger problems, too, is essential. How severely traumatised are the patients? Are their problems complex in nature?

We neither set store by nor reject specific treatment methods. Many different methods are effective, provided the therapist has a solid foundation of high-quality training. One of the best methods at therapists' disposal may be body-oriented. The more severely traumatised the patient is, the more important the therapist's knowledge of trauma and dissociation becomes. Severe trauma calls for a more comprehensive assessment.

For complex traumatisation and more severe syndromes, the treatment needs to be based on a multi-phase or multi-stage process. The phase-oriented process we advocate includes trauma-related dissociation and provides scope for many different methods of treatment to be applied, when necessary, to achieve specific purposes. The more complex the traumatisation, the greater the need to work using an integrative approach of this kind. This approach, in our view, provides a sufficiently open basis for seeing the individual variations.

Three phases

The degree of traumatisation determines the work procedure. Guiding a patient to visit a trauma memory in the body, without the therapist knowing much about the content of the trauma, may work fine. But the more severe the dissociative syndrome, the more essential it is to have a wealth of knowledge about the patient so as to know when, where and how exposure to such a memory can be done.

Treatment of severe mental traumatisation may be divided into the following three stages.

1. Stabilise

Trauma therapy needs to begin with the stabilisation phase — a precondition for the trauma itself to be treatable. In this phase, patients' ability to understand their own reactions and manage their feelings is strengthened. There are countless practical techniques, in the form of physical and psychological exercises, mental training, and much more, that survivors can learn. They can then use them to empower themselves to stay in their own bodies and attain balance.

2. Focus on the trauma

Together, in the next stage, the patient and the therapist review the traumatising events. Trauma-focused treatment always involves some form of exposure, when patients encounter and relives their own traumatic experiences. Here, the proper balance between work and rest is important. A reasonable pace is necessary, and space must be allowed for insights, recovery and mourning.

3. Integrate

The third phase is a matter of reorientation. Patients are helped to integrate the trauma as part of their own story and move on in life, so that they are no longer ruled by fear and a destructive self-image.

Before starting treatment, the therapist thus has to find out how traumatised the person is. Does the problem consist in post-traumatic stress disorder (PTSD) or perhaps an even more severe form of traumatisation, such as dissociative identity disorder (DID)?

The professional may think it is ordinary, simple PTSD and begin treatment for this when the patient is actually suffering from complex PTSD or a more severe dissociative disorder. If this happens, the treatment can damage the individual if the traumatising events start being relived and processed too early on. Integration needs to be preceded by a thorough stabilisation phase.

Chapter 13 explores phase-oriented trauma-focused psychotherapy in more detail.

Traumatisation hard to measure

By means of an interview, self-assessment scales and a clinical assessment, the extent of a person's traumatisation can be gauged. If the patient's self-assessment scales show a high degree of dissociative symptoms, the therapist needs to conduct a manual-based interview to get a thorough grasp of the degree of dissociation. The professional needs subtle discernment to carry out this kind of interview and make correct assessments.

When professionals assess psychological suffering, they tend to use established terminology. In psychiatry, the predominant systems are the *Diagnostic and Statistical Manual of Mental Disorders* (DSM) and the *International Classification of Diseases* (ICD). All 'mental disorders' are classified according to these two diagnostic systems. Both are blunt assessment tools and inadequate for understanding people. Nonetheless, an attempt to identify the degree of traumatisation, in order to determine the treatment focus, is important. The DSM system does not distinguish between simple PTSD and complex PTSD. ICD — the World Health Organisation's (WHO) international statistical classification system of diagnostic codes — is now the first system to suggest giving complex post-traumatic stress disorder a separate designation in the version ICD-11. This may help clarification on diagnoses, treatment and research on trauma.

People's experiences and difficulties can never really, of course, be placed in systems of square pigeonholes.

Trauma-related dissociative disorder

> ### *Dissociation*
>
> *A collective term for numerous different symptoms. In its most severe form, 'structural dissociation', the outcome has been fragmentation, which means a disintegration of the personality into two or more dissociative parts that exist in one and the same person.*

Chapter 7 ('Attachment system: the necessary bonds') was about our attachment patterns, which are shaped in early childhood. These unconscious patterns characterise us far into adulthood and are crucial in determining how traumatic experiences affect us.

People of a trusting nature, who have formed secure attachment, are best equipped to deal with difficult experiences. When a person who suffers from severe trauma has an underlying pattern of insecure attachment, on the other hand, the consequences are worse, and this person risks developing a greater degree of traumatisation. For those with insecure-avoidant or insecure-ambivalent attachment patterns, the risk of developing complex PTSD is also higher. In a disorganised attachment pattern, the person not infrequently develops 'trauma-related structural dissociation'.

In such cases, the severely traumatising situations have been numerous and recurrent, often taking place over a long period after starting an early age. If the victim is subjected continuously to such situations, perhaps even to abuse by an adult in the child's immediate vicinity — people who are really supposed to be kind and provide good care — then there are high risks that the disorder will be of the severest kind.

Red alert

A disorganised attachment pattern results in a life crammed with perceptions of chaos. Nothing is secure, nothing feels trustworthy or safe — least of all the person's inner self. Thoughts, feelings and bodily sensations rush around, in an existence often dominated by the defence system.

Individuals struggle to master and live their lives, based on their age and life situation. Sometimes, professionals get involved and these people get help and adequate treatment. Sometimes, unfortunately, nothing comes of this. They create strategies to master their existence as best they can, but are not infrequently defeated by the task. When life goes on and their everyday existence no longer consists of threatening situations, the internal chaos nonetheless persists. Echoes from their childhood fill the present and they are trapped in profound insecurity. Disasters lie constantly in wait and the person lives at the highest alert level. The period of the traumatic experiences has ended, although emotional parts of the personality do not understand this. Parts in the individual have 'frozen' in the past and remain in the state of perceiving threats, constantly on red alert.

Traumatised people are thus somewhere on the trauma spectrum, with their own degree of traumatisation. What is known as simple PTSD is the mildest degree of injury. If there were deficiencies in basic security during childhood and the attachment patterns have become insecure, the child's vulnerability increases. If children suffer painful events at an early age without being helped to handle their reactions, the risk of traumatisation rises. If the events are also recurrent and children have the misfortune to be continuously exposed to neglect or abuse, perhaps even at the hands of adults in their immediate surroundings, the danger of complex PTSD increases.

A severe, trauma-related dissociative disorder affects people only if they have been exposed to repeated trauma at an early age. There is no precise research regarding age, but 'early' is usually considered to be before the child is six to eight years old. Experiencing extreme neglect and abuse in early life can lead to exceptionally complex states known as structural dissociation.

More details about the trauma scale, and of the various states of traumatisation, are given at the end of this book. Let us now look further at what happens in the brain and body when trauma leads to dissociation.

Shrinking hippocampus

When we experience something threatening, many things happen in our bodies and the brain goes into overdrive. The body signals danger. The heart beats faster, the pulse quickens and there is a rush of adrenaline. The brain tries to grasp the situation and decide what survival requires. But the traumatised brain cannot work out how to deal with the danger. The information process seizes up, disconnecting the speech network.

Today, we know that repeated traumatic events can alter brain structure. For example, they change the size of the hippocampus — the region that helps to orient us and our memories in time and space. There are studies showing that in people with the most severe dissociative disorder, 'DID', the hippocampus has shrunk by 25 per cent. The good news is that, in those affected, the hippocampus has grown back to normal size after successful psychotherapeutic treatment.

A dissociative failure of personality integration may thus arise because people's stress management system is overwhelmed by what happens to them. Children subjected to such incidents cannot then integrate their perceptions and feelings. The victim is unable to transform these experiences into events that have taken place in the past but are now over and done with. The horrific memories lack context. There is no means of emotion regulation, nor can inner serenity emerge.

Greatly simplified, the defence system may be said to be regulated in a primitive part of the brain and its branches. This region becomes underactive in states of dissociation. If this occurs repeatedly from an early age, several distinct parts of the personality may arise. Each of these may carry certain painful memories and create various patterns and behaviours in an effort to survive.

In the traumatised brain, the memory fails to reach the prefrontal cortex — that is, the part of the brain that normally helps us deal with changes. Without a functioning prefrontal cortex, we cannot understand what we feel and why. When terrifying recollections dominate and live a life of their own, we can no longer control our own bodies.

Fragmented inner world

Thus, structural dissociation does not mean that the personality 'breaks' or divides into several parts, like a vase that falls on the floor and shatters into a thousand pieces. Rather, a coherent adult personality never develops. The vase has never been shaped by soft caring hands, nurtured into being during childhood. Small children are entirely absorbed in their experiences and ruled by their feelings. Different aspects of the personality are formed during the child's various development stages. When this process is disturbed, these parts of the person do not merge: the child's consciousness of being a single person never arises, and integration into a coherent self fails to take place.

Structural dissociation is often caused by repeated threatening events. Something that never should happen in a child's life occurs over and over again. The lack of interconnectedness among the child's various parts may also be due to something failing to occur: something that *should* happen. The necessary attention or affirmation, or the crucial warmth, care and understanding, is not provided. Nor do such children get help in interpreting sensory perceptions, whether their own or other people's. Instead, small children like this are left abandoned in their own fragmented emotional world, which fails to fuse together as they grow up.

No interconnection

When the interconnecting process is inadequate or entirely absent, or emerges in a threatening environment, small 'islands' may be created. Several 'emotional parts of the personality' arise. The individual inner person becomes like an orchestra without a conductor. Each instrument plays its own melody, at its own tempo and in its own world. With no unity or coordination, the music sounds chaotic.

Each separate part of the individual sees itself as an entity requiring self-defence. Each carries different memories and can remember completely different events. Memory gaps are frequent. One part is unaware, or only vaguely aware, of what happened while another was in charge. What the different parts know about their multiplicity and the passing of time varies. They differ in what they focus their attention on and seek to achieve. They may be dominated by differing reaction patterns from the defence system. Similarly, the nature of their attachment patterns may change to some extent.

A minor, vulnerable and fearful emotional part may, for example, have a very strong bond with the perpetrator. A desire to be obliging, or not to be noticed, may be highly dominant. Within moments, another emotional part may come to the fore. Ruled by a need for control and self-defence, this part acts in anger and with overwhelmingly strong resistance if anyone is perceived as intrusive. Each part may perceive the world on the basis of the child's age when it developed.

These inner parts are often described by trauma survivors as incapable of cooperating. One common perception is that dissociative parts often 'lose time' and do not know what has happened. They may arrive at a place without knowing how they got there. Sometimes they do not recognise family members or friends, or they may have the sense that their own body does not belong to them. They discover that they behave very differently in similar situations, as if they were completely separate people.

Ego states and parts of the personality

Sometimes the term 'dissociative part of the personality' is used when what is actually meant is an 'ego state'. Awareness of the difference is important.

A healthy person — who has no problems of dissociation — may struggle with ambivalence and conflicting desires, and even different ego states that are not well integrated. But these ego states all sail under one and the same flag. They are subject to joint command and control. Thus, they are not at all the same as the phenomenon of dissociative parts of the personality that characterise a person with a dissociative syndrome. A dissociative personality is divided into considerably more clearly demarcated parts, which all have their own sense of who they are, what the world is like and how they relate to others.

Sometimes these concepts create confusion among therapists and other clinicians. The difference between ego states and dissociative parts of the personality is blurred or not understood. Teachers in the area of therapy testify that many students contend with confusion due to conflicting definitions in the trauma literature. The concepts thus need clarifying.

People who suffer from trauma-related dissociation have often had highly dramatic experiences. One example is a male patient, one of whose emotional parts was still in prison and being tortured, although it was several years since the man had been released and left his home country. As a result, he had major difficulties in everyday life. He was unable to look at himself in a mirror without the mirror image becoming the prison guard who had tortured him. Consequently, the man was unable to use most lavatories.

Another problem was that he could not always move his body as he wanted, because his emotional part was still tied up with rope. He was unable to shake hands, because his hands were tied behind his back. One minute, he might speak lovingly about his mother and younger siblings; moments later, he understood no Swedish at all, had a desperate look in his eyes and just wanted to escape. He often relived the gruesome torture he had experienced, and tried to use his hands to protect his body from the fire, the screws and the weights on his genitals. To get to therapy he would travel one stop at a time, stepping off at each underground station because of his fear and confusion. Not infrequently, he got lost and travelled in the wrong direction.

Locked in a dark wardrobe

One woman had an emotional part of her personality who thought she was four years old. She lived in a dark wardrobe and greatly feared light. This was linked to memories of having been shut in a wardrobe, unsure when anyone would open the door next, and never knowing whether it would mean getting some food or being subjected to new violent abuse. When the four-year-old part was in charge, she would crawl into a corner of the treatment room, sucking her thumb. It was then hard to understand what she was saying, if indeed she said anything at all.

Sometimes, she just sat and shook forcefully; sometimes she whispered in a very weak, childlike voice, *'Was I wrong? Sorry, Mum... sorry... no... no...'* Once, in the present, she sat in the same corner of her flat for eight days. Later, the woman said she had been unable to move, as if completely paralysed. She knew she had to stay completely still because she had previously been naughty and noisy.

All these upsetting situations in the present, both for the formerly tortured man and for the woman who had been locked up in childhood, arose because different parts in them took command at various times. These emotional parts of their personalities were quite different from ego states in a healthy, integrated person with conflicting desires.

It is extremely important to find out the extent of the trauma every individual bears. What can help this person, in particular? Are there two or more parts of the personality that need to be invited into the therapy? A thorough assessment is crucial.

We now meet Yasmine. Even as a young child, she was raped, abused and maltreated. Horror and powerlessness are her companions. Her road to a healthy life is long and arduous.

FOURTH STORY

Yasmine is referred to TT by a doctor. At first, she is too weak to climb the stairs. It turns out that she is taking huge amounts of medication. She is drugged, in a very poor state, and has undergone many electroconvulsive treatments. She does not want to live and says her whole life is chaos. Yasmine has been a psychiatric inpatient for many months, repeatedly. She has been on sick leave for a long time and is unable to cope with being a mother to her children.

That first session is the starting point for prolonged therapeutic treatment. When her therapy is completed several years later, among the last things she says is how very grateful she is and how she now has just one wish left: to do something for other trauma victims. Yasmine wants to tell her story, and hopes it may help someone.

Yasmine's wish sows the first seed for this book.

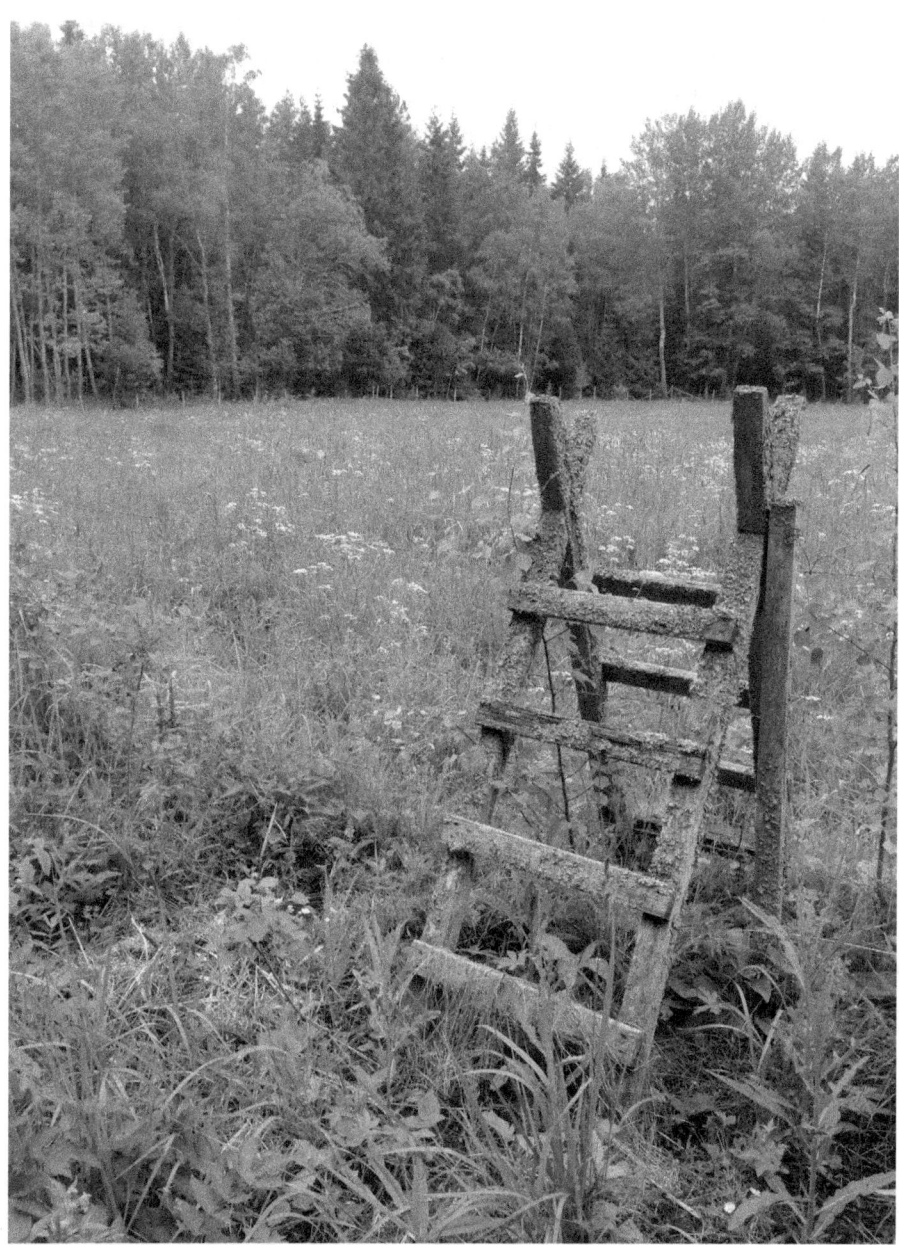

By Annica Lilja Ljung

Yasmine

Sexual abuse, deficient care, adults' betrayal and grief for siblings who have taken their own lives cause Yasmine's personality to split into several dissociative parts.

'I've lost a lot: my childhood, my siblings, my life… I end up in a mental hospital, pumped full of pills, and have 52 electric shock treatments. Nobody listens to me.'

The way my life is now is completely different: there's no comparison. Now I'm very happy and positive. Before, I was terribly depressed. I was a prisoner inside myself. I never believed that one day I might be able to work and feel well.

Four or five years ago, I had no life. All I wanted was to leave this world. My life meant nothing. I wanted love, but just felt disgusting and was afraid of closeness.

Happily running around

I grew up in Thailand with four siblings. Now I only have one left. It feels like I didn't have any childhood. No, I don't know what being a child is like. I never got the chance.

My friends played, but I had to work and be a good girl. Mum wanted help with the cooking and I had to look after my two little sisters as well. I was like an extra mother. Always busy, to avoid feeling.

When I saw the other children playing, I wondered how it would feel to run around like that, happy and free. I was never able to be myself as a child. Now, looking back, I understand how that went on affecting me, constantly. That's all my parents were capable of. I suppose they did what they could.

My body was so thin you could count the ribs. Skinny as a rake, I carried my little sister around on my hip. She had no nappy, so I got dirty. It was disgusting.

While I was looking after the younger children, they sometimes fell asleep by my side. Then I fell asleep too. I was tired. I was often woken up by a slap. I was beaten when I'd done wrong. I was constantly afraid of being punished, and tried to defend myself and get away.

When Dad and Mum slaughtered chickens I'd pluck the feathers and clean out everything inside that could be sold. When I was five, I had to learn how to sell chickens in the market, which began early in the morning. To be in place by four o'clock, I was woken up in the middle of the night — one in the morning.

But now I'll try to tell you about the really painful thing: the abuse by my father.

Holding hands

When I'm six years old, Dad comes in to me at night to rape me. He grabs my body and forces his way into me. It hurts so much that I scream. Then Dad holds my mouth. I'm stiff with terror.

My sister and I sleep in the same room. She's 13, I think. Already, I've seen and heard Dad raping my sister. I was scared, but didn't understand what was happening. Now he attacks me too.

I'm six years old when it starts. Dad smells revoltingly of cigarette smoke. His voice is like a monster's. I cry and cry. Close my eyes. Don't want to see, don't want to be there. My sister cries too. She can't help me.

We usually hold hands when Dad comes into our room to force himself on her or me. Every morning after Dad has been on me, she plaits my hair to console me. But she says nothing.

I know nothing else. So I think Dad's love is normal. But why, then, is it so painful? And why does Dad say I can't talk to anyone about what he does to us?

Does love hurt?

Dad rapes us often. Although I'm still in pain after the last time, he thrusts himself into me again. He hurts me. The pain is terrible and never-ending. It lasts for ever. I'm so lonely there in the dark. So scared. So small and vulnerable.

Dad says it's love — that he loves me. But if that's love, I don't want any of it. So I shut myself off. Don't want to feel anything. Just want it to end. I become like a hard stone. I feel so empty. All the familiar sounds that usually surround me as I lie in bed in the evening — barking dogs, clucking chickens, cackling hens — are gone. I hear nothing. I'm not there.

In Thailand, child-beating is allowed. Dad thrashes me hard on my body and legs with a stick when he's angry. One day he hits me so hard on the head that I faint. If I haven't finished getting a meal on time, he kicks me. Then I get no food. I go hungry. If he doesn't think the food tastes good, I have to start from scratch and cook a new meal.

Disgusting me

Dad says terrible things. He says I'm bad. That I'm the worst. That I'm disgusting. Everyone in the village knows I'm useless. He often says: *'She's crazy! She's disobedient!'* Then nobody wants to be with me. Our neighbours don't want their children to play with me.

I'm ashamed. Feel confused and helpless. Dirty, disgusting and terribly lonely.

My fingers are black from all the work. I'm envious of girls who have soft hands with clean nails. I'm never clean. I'm just disgusting. I'm bullied at school. They hold their noses and say I smell bad. Then I get sad. It feels like everyone hates me. I know I smell of pee and keep away. Don't like myself at all.

All of us siblings, and Mum too, are afraid of Dad. We know we'll be punished. We're never safe. So we obey him. Don't dare do anything else.

Dad decides everything and forces me to do what he says. I do whatever Dad wants, as best I can, but he's never satisfied. Everything I do is wrong. In his eyes, I'm a worthless little human being. He never sees what I need, and he oversteps every limit.

My beloved sister

Mum just cries and cries. She doesn't dare say anything when Dad's bad. He often beats her. In our culture, the wife doesn't leave her husband. She stays with him. Instead of protecting me and my siblings, Mum drinks spirits. She never talks about what Dad does to me and my sister at night. After Dad has been mean, she says nothing about what's taken place, as if it has never happened.

Dad says *'I love you'* to my sister. Then he does that terrible thing to her that hurts so much. I feel that she's in a really bad way. We get extremely close to each other. But she doesn't want me to see when she's sad, so she wipes away the tears. She shows me that you have to be strong.

One day when my sister's 14, I see that her eyes are terribly sad. I follow her like a shadow. Then she goes into another room and says I can't come in. I *want* to follow her, but she says no. I sense something's wrong, so I sit on the floor outside the closed door and wait. After a while I hear BANG! I run in and see that my sister has shot herself in the head. I stand there, only seven years old, and know why she did it. Dad had tried to sell her on the street as a sex slave. She prefers to die. The walls are spattered with her blood. That sight is stuck on my retina forever.

I know, but don't understand. *How can my sister just leave me? Why does she do this to me? Why is she abandoning me?*

It's hard to grasp that she's gone. At night, I imagine her smell and the feel of her hand. And I cry out in the dark: *'You're here, aren't you?'* But I get no answer.

Heart-breaking

After my sister's suicide, Dad comes to me all the time and takes me by force. I don't understand what's happening and think it's normal — that all fathers do that. He says I've got to keep quiet about it, and nobody will believe me if I tell them. The villagers will say I'm crazy. I know Dad's good at talking and lying so that people believe him, so I keep quiet.

To have the strength to work and be good, I take painkillers. I switch off the awful things. I fear Dad's anger even more strongly than I fear the pain.

Mum knows what's happening. She starts drinking even more. Escapes into intoxication. Drinks until she vomits. Falls asleep. Lets me down. My maternal grandmother probably understands what's happening to her grandchild, because she starts drinking too. In the end, Gran can't take it any longer. Using pills, she takes her own life. And my cousin does the same. I think her father too wants to sell her on the street and make money. She takes medicine as well, so then she's gone from my life as well.

My sister, grandmother, cousin… so many dead people. It's too much for me to bear. Slowly but surely, my heart breaks.

I long terribly for my big sister. One day I suddenly step straight out into the street in front of a motorbike. After the impact, I lie unconscious in hospital for days. When I wake up, I cry in despair. Why haven't I succeeded like my sister? I want to get away from Dad, to escape, just as she's done. And I want to go to her. It doesn't matter whether it's in heaven or hell, as long as I can be with my sister.

My brother and me

I feel safe at the hospital. The nurses are so nice. I want to stay there, but have to go back.

Back at home, the violence goes on. My big brother may beat me at any time. Our father teaches him it's okay. One day, Dad forces my brother to have sex with me: him, Dad and me, all three together. Dad tells him that guys have the power and girls are nothing. He forces my brother to do what he does himself. Nobody dares defy him.

Waiting for night to come feels like a nightmare. I'm not allowed to leave the house. I can't talk to anyone and describe how scared I am. I have no friend, no mother, to listen.

I have every reason to be angry but am not allowed to be. I feel emotionally cut off. Nobody understands me. So I often sit in the cool shade under my favourite tree and talk to my 'friends'. They exist only there. I don't know how they come to me, but I sort of split myself into several people. There's a little one called Sara. One who's angry — that's Tana. And then me, the everyday girl Yasmine. There are three of us voices inside me, three different people. I really believe it *is* like that! No one else notices anything and I don't dare tell. But my 'friends' understand and usually wish me well.

Freedom inside me

Sometimes we disagree. Tana wants to argue with Dad and everyone else. She gets angry with Sara and me, but it's mostly me she scolds and shouts at. Still, with Tana and Sara I find a little, tiny bit of security. They give me a feeling of freedom inside. Afterwards, I realise it's Little Sara who stepped out into the street and then wanted to stay in hospital.

I'm not really supposed to sit there under the tree, in my own world. I should be at home, working. But now there are several of us, I dare to disobey. We support one another. *'Now we'll get a beating when we get home, but we can take that,'* one voice says out loud. The others feel the blows and the pain just like me. They're afraid just as I am. Now I'm not alone any longer and that feels wonderful. I don't really understand it, but feel it's helping me.

I can't flee the assaults or escape from my body. There's no way out. But my friends help me escape into myself. With them, I find some comfort and security. I feel they really exist in me and are helping me. Now I don't have to be alone any more. When I'm down, I talk to them and hear their voices. I can trust my friends. Without them I won't survive.

Dad sells my body

The first time I get my female period, I don't understand a thing. Warm blood runs down my legs. I get a shock. I know nothing about my body.

When I'm 13 or 14, Dad thinks it's time for me to bring in money. I'm pretty and slim. He sells me on the street to foreign tourists. Every day for over a year I'm sold as a prostitute in Pattaya. Because I'm so young, he can sell me several times a day.

My body's invaded. The pain... the terror... the powerlessness... it's impossible to describe how it feels. Words aren't enough.

I remember the pain in my genitals. How they bleed every day. How tired and sad I am. A doctor tries to stop the assaults. He tells Dad I'm injured and have to rest. But Dad doesn't care about that.

My brother raped me for several years. Suddenly, Dad starts selling him, too, to tourists who want sex. Then, something happens in my brother. He doesn't want to have sex with me any more and he no longer hits me. My brother is kind to me. When I get home, he's sitting there, waiting for me. He greets me with a warm smile, and has bought something tasty for me to eat — something he know I like. It's brotherly love, for real.

Being sold to strange men for sex is a dreadful thing. One day when I'm sitting and waiting for my brother, I suddenly hear a terrified scream. I rush there and see my brother hanging, dead, with horribly staring eyes. I'll never forget that sight. In despair, I yell: *'You're betraying me too, just like our sister!'*

How can I accept his death? Now I'm more alone than ever, but my 'friends' are still alive. Today I know my brother couldn't take it any longer. I can understand him.

Unknown men

Dad continues to sell me to male strangers — always Westerners. I don't understand any English and can't make myself understood. I feel vulnerable. My prostitution brings in lots of money, but I can't understand where it goes. I don't want to realise that my parents are gambling away the money. But one day when I come home after a rough night, a man at the bar says Mum and Dad have a big debt to him. That's why they're selling my body.

I hate men. I hate the fact that it's impossible to wash away all that repulsiveness. To make life bearable, I shut down all my feelings. I become numb, paralysed. I escape inwards, to my invisible friends that I've split into. They aren't make-believe friends. They really exist. Now I myself start to think I am crazy, just as Dad says. So I don't tell anyone.

Confused

Being several people feels great. I can tell them exactly how things are without having to fear being beaten. Tana struggles hard. She knows everything that's happened and is subjected to the abuse just like me. We want to believe Sara is an innocent girl. We see her playing carefreely. When Sara can't hear, we tell each other that nothing nasty has happened in her world. Meanwhile I, Yasmine, diligently struggle on. I talk to others, go to school and do my everyday duties. I don't dare do anything else. Tana and I want to protect little Sara and save her from the truth.

Sara can be free. She gets to play and be a child, as I've never been allowed to be. I make her a doll out of palm leaves to make her happy.

One morning, I wake up with bruises on my body. I'm surprised and have no idea what's happened. When I ask Tana, she tells me she quarrelled with Dad. She protested and then he beat her. Tana thinks I'm a coward. That's why she defends me and Sara. I don't know anything about her fight with Dad. I never know anything about it, but maybe that's why Dad calls me unruly — me, the one who never dares say anything against him!

Sold to Sweden

When I'm 16, Dad sells me to an older man, who takes me to Sweden. The passport says I'm 20, but it isn't true. They make me out to be an adult although I'm a child and send me away — abroad, far away.

The man who buys me is 49 years old. Sweden is cold. Snow is peculiar stuff. I can't talk to him and don't know where I've ended up.

My husband is violent. He threatens and abuses, hits and rapes me. I'm very sad. He throws things at me and tells me to leave. My suitcase is hurled through the air at me. He wants to throw me out. But I have no money and no relative to turn to. I don't know any Swedish, speak English badly and don't know how Sweden works. *Where should I go?* I'm so alone and scared. So I kneel down and plead, sobbing, *'Please, please let me stay!'* His power over me is total. I'm isolated, feel disgusting and blame myself. When I have a baby daughter, he doesn't let me breastfeed, gets jealous and doesn't want me to go near her.

Neither Sara nor Tana want to be with him. I explain to them that we must. We just have to grit our teeth and bear it. Little Sara is terrified and wants to hide. Tana is furious. I struggle to keep all the painful feelings in check.

When we visit Thailand, my husband leaves me with my parents to go out and buy young girls. Then he infects me with sexually transmitted diseases.

Who am I?

At home in Sweden, I start working at a factory. My husband takes from me every penny I earn, but I make friends at work and feel a little stronger. I want to get away from him, but he threatens me. When I meet a guy who works at the same place, he helps me make the break.

In the divorce, I get nothing. My husband has arranged a prenuptial agreement. Everything is his: the house, the boat, even the plot of land in Thailand. With my parents' help, he has faked my signature. So I don't get a thing. But I don't care about the money, as long as I get away from the arguments.

I move in with my workmate. He's kind, but I feel no love. My daughter lives with us. Soon we have a baby together. Life is hard. I'm young and confused. I don't know who I am and have never learnt what love is. When I get pregnant again after a couple of years, he forces me to have an abortion. Then I want to leave him. There's a very strong feeling inside me: *I can't trust anyone who wants to kill my child.* The angry part of me gives me the strength to break up. She says, *'Come on, it's time to move. We can't live with a man who takes his own child's life.'*

My partner keeps the apartment and our daughter stays with him. Leaving my child hurts very much, but I move out anyway. I live alone with my eldest daughter. All the time, I save money to be able to send it to my parents and siblings. Tana protests. We can never agree on that. She wants us to keep the money. But I explain that we have to help my little siblings and my poor grandfather at home in Thailand. She agrees to that.

A new life

Tana helps me a lot. She learns how society works in Sweden, and struggles to learn Swedish and find out about her rights. She's tough when I'm cowardly. She dares to argue. Without her, I'd never have managed — I see that now.

I survive by trying to forget about the assaults and keep all painful memories away. I switch off, and shut them deep inside me.

After a while I meet Magnus, who I've now lived with for 18 years. We're married and have two children together. For the first few months, he comes and goes as he likes. Then he asks: *'Would you like to move in with me?'*

Magnus is 31 when we meet. I'm 35. With him, I try to get on with my life. When we have a baby boy, we're thrilled. Seeing his face is an indescribable joy. Magnus is so happy when he carries our newborn baby around. He changes his nappies, bathes him and is really nice.

I'm overwhelmed. I've never seen a man like that before. I feel like a queen, but sometimes I'm envious of the child. After all, I've never had a good Dad.

I think I'm crazy

We have another baby. I stay home with the children for more than a decade. My husband supports us. I feel love, but sometimes my husband sees flashes of hate in my eyes. I'm so *angry* in my whole body, I can't speak. Neither my husband nor I understand what's happening, but it's as if I'm living in the past. When my husband sees my hateful look, it's about the hatred of all the other men, the ones who've hurt me.

When our youngest child is six, I start working. It feels like I'm working 24 hours a day. I look after our home and children, and then work in the home care service in the evening while the children sleep. At weekends, I do double shifts. I never have time to rest, nor ever to calm down.

It's hard to say who decides I have to work so much. But I simply can't say no when they call and ask me to come. How do you say no? I don't know. Ever since early childhood, I've learnt to be submissive and useful to others, to have no control, not to feel my limits. Never to say '*Stop.*'

When I change jobs, it gets even worse. Finally, my head just goes BANG. My brain can't take it any more, and stops working. It's like blowing a fuse. Chaos. My memory doesn't work at all.

I don't remember what happened, but I end up in hospital. For several years I'm more or less out of this world. Three or four years just disappear. When I finally start waking up, I find it hard to believe that it's really true. It's difficult to explain, but when you end up in a psychiatric clinic, it feels like everything gets even worse. Then I really believe I'm crazy.

Nobody listens

The wounds from childhood catch up with me. I don't have the strength to be a mother. I'm not capable of showing love to my children, or giving them what they needed. I don't dare fall asleep for fear of all the terrible memories coming back. I go in and out of the hospital's high-security inpatient units and get masses of pills. I can't speak. My mouth feels heavy and I just do as they say.

Finally, I'm totally out of it, and remember nothing. No one understands what's wrong. I long for love but can't express it. I don't have the strength to live. The doctors give me 52 electric shock treatments (ECT). Nothing helps.

At the psychiatric clinic, I try to say that there are several parts of me, and talk about my parts. But nobody listens. They don't understand that I need something different from drugs and ECT. I try to explain: *'I'm not just me. I'm several people.'* They treat me as if I'm insane and have sick fantasies. It feels like the doctors don't know that people can be in that situation, with several people inside them. Finally, I give up. Would you have the strength to tell someone again and again that you're three people, without being believed? No. So you don't have the strength to keep talking.

Pills and ECT

To get attention, I cut myself. It's my way of shouting *'Listen to me! Hug me! I need you now!'* I'm in a rage and argue with everyone. I can't say what I need, and the staff don't understand. All I want is for someone to understand and help me when I'm so sad and hurt. Instead, they lock me up. Then I really think I've gone crazy. I want to vanish from it all. Take my life.

I get loads of medication and ECT. The treatment destroys me, and gives me epilepsy. It feels like everyone hates me. When they see me shaking with anxiety, they say, *'Here — take the pill.'* But that doesn't change anything. I'm still split into several parts. The awful things come back, and I feel like a prisoner. To prevent me injuring myself, I have to lie strapped down on my bed.

One part of me no longer wants to live. She can't bear the anxiety and pain in my body. *'Now let's stop living like this,'* she says, and wants me to throw myself in front of the Metro train. But another part of me puts a stop to it.

When I cut myself, I see the wound and the blood, but don't feel the pain. I want it to hurt, so that I forget the pain in my soul. But I feel nothing. The nurse is even able to stitch me up without an anaesthetic. My heartache is bad. I feel like taking a whole container of tranquillisers to avoid feeling anything.

Witch's rage

Since I'm very ill, Magnus and the children don't have an easy time. I can't face responsibility. The scars on the inside of my wrists are bright red. On some days I'm nice, on others a wicked witch. I get angry about the tiniest thing. The whole bathroom cabinet is full of my medicines. I'm carrying a powerful rage, a great protest inside me.

Tana can really *hate*. She and I have to protect Sara. She's a virgin and isn't noticed that much. If someone gets too close to Sara, we push him away.

During that time, I can be furious at my husband for three or four days but can't say why.

My husband has to take a lot of crap. Yelling, mean words, the lot! He puts up with everything. Throughout the storm, he stands his ground. He has tremendous patience.

Thank goodness I get referred to TT. Today I know I was in touch with her for several years, but for me it feels like just a few months. Isn't that strange?

No longer disgusting

I'm lucky. I get to see TT once a week, and for a while even twice a week. She talks to me, listens carefully and sees my inner world. In the beginning, I find it hard to trust her. There's so much anger in my body. The terror and rage are in the whole of me. I don't let her too close. I test her, and I'm on my guard. Still, I want to go back there.

I've felt really disgusting, as if everything I've been through is my own fault. That's why I've been so afraid to tell anyone what I've been through — to show who I am. I've been convinced that my husband and everyone else would think I was disgusting. I thought no one would want to get close to me if they knew. But seeing TT gives me hope; this is something completely new. She looks me in the eyes and says, *'You're not crazy.'*

It takes time to create the trust that's needed to become secure. *Maybe she's just being kind because she's getting paid.* Slowly, my confidence in her grows. I tell her what I've been through and cry a lot. Every time, the anxiety is almost unbearable, but I always feel better afterwards. In the end, I dare to feel I really want a hug from her, and even dare ask for it. When she hugs me, I begin to realise I'm not disgusting… and finally I don't feel disgusting any more.

Where am I going?

At first, I'm afraid TT will think I'm weird being several people. I think maybe I won't be allowed to keep seeing her if she gets to know that there are several of me. But it's the opposite. She definitely wants me to continue in therapy.

Sometimes one part of my personality totally takes over, without me knowing. It may be for a short while, but also for several days. Tana, for instance, can go shopping and spend masses of money. Afterwards, I can't remember anything.

On my way home from therapy, I can suddenly switch to another person. I kind of disappear from my own sight. When I come to, I don't know where I am or where I'm going. I can wake up on the bus or somewhere else without having a clue how I've got there. Then I have to ask strangers, *'Excuse me, where am I?'* I ask the bus driver: *'How long have I been travelling with you?'* He gives me a really strange look. Then I feel ashamed.

I used to think this had happened only to me. The abuse. The anxiety. Being in several parts. The confusion. I felt like the loneliest person in the world and lived with my secrets. Now I understand that other people suffer like that too. When I think about the fact that we're many, that it's not just me, the shame lets me go.

Lovely liberation

TT helps me develop the communication among all the parts of my personality. They've been there the whole time, but now it's steadily getting clearer how we work and don't work together. We're always pulling in different directions, and have different answers to most questions. It feels awkward when she starts poking into my secrets, but at the same time a great relief. Like a liberation. I begin to realise that all the parts are me!

We go carefully, coaxing them out one by one and asking whether they want to appear. It can take a long time before a part dares to show herself — before she trusts that it's safe.

The Angry One can appear at any time in daily life. She always says what she thinks, and I can't stop her. She's still back there, in the old days. Still angry. She thinks TT is clueless and wants to argue with her, like a teenager.

Living with many different parts of myself is really hard work, especially when they're at loggerheads. Tana doesn't want to have therapy at all. She makes a fuss and tries to slink away. But it doesn't work: TT is too steady and strong. She doesn't let us down. She gets Tana to agree to come, and suddenly Tana too is working hard in the therapy. I don't really know how TT gets her to do it, but then it happens a lot.

Scared little Sara

To start with, I don't let little Sara come to the therapy. She doesn't like being left alone at home, but Tana and I don't think she's experienced the rapes, and want to protect her from the truth. So we join forces and decide not to let her come with us to TT. Little Sara has to stay at home and play with the children's toys. Finally, we accept the idea of taking her to TT. Then we — adult, everyday Yasmine and angry Tana — realise that Sara, the nice little girl, has been there too when Dad came at night. At first we're truly horrified, then just surprised. It takes a long time to understand.

It feels so good for Sara to be allowed to join in at last. She who is so young lives on in the old present: in our childhood. Alone and scared. TT coaxes her out in the therapy room by buying a small, soft rabbit toy that she can hug and cuddle. She's always wanted a soft animal toy and has never been allowed to be a secure child. Now she can play. Slowly, slowly she calms down and eventually feels safe.

I haven't been allowed to be angry either. To set any limits, or say no. Now Tana makes a stubborn fuss. She says she doesn't want to. She shouts, *'You're lying!'* when TT says she really thinks we'll get well and find a job. I can't really believe she means it either. But she goes on believing in me.

Sometimes I get cramp in my stomach when I go to the therapy. I just want to get out of going there. I get so angry that I feel feverish. When I arrive there, everything feels like hard going. It only takes about a minute for the whole world to fall apart. My body shakes. It feels like I was going to die. But I have to face all the awfulness. It has to be let out. Afterwards, it's a tremendous relief.

All three are me

We work extremely hard. TT talks to all three of us. No one has ever done that before. I, Yasmine, was the one who talked to the others. After a while, two different parts can meet and begin understanding each other. In the end, the parts of my personality talk to one another about the difficult stuff. They begin to grasp that the danger is over, that Dad can't hurt me any longer. Before they understood one another, they weren't really able to cooperate. Now they see eye to eye.

We are really different. We have different thoughts, wishes and feelings, and completely different perceptions of our body. For a long time we also have different dreams, but finally I start to think: *Who is TT really talking to? It's* me *answering every time!* In wonder, I realise that everyone is me: Tana, the strong one who struggles; scared little Sara who wants to be allowed to play and be secure; and the adult, everyday Yasmine. *Can they all be me?* Now I begin getting the feeling... that it's like coming home. First Yasmine and Tana are occasionally getting close, really close. Then the occasions gradually lengthen.

When I wake up one morning, the parts of my personality tell one another what they have dreamt during the night. It turns out they've all had the same dream! Before, Tana used to talk about a horrible dream she'd had during the night, but the others didn't understand a thing. Now, we've all experienced the same dream. Dreamt the same thing!

Facing terror in security

Through the therapy, I wake up to my life. I hardly remember anything about the time when my children were little. Now I want time to go backwards so that I can give them love early in life. But it's too late. We have to live with it as it is. It hurts to realise that my daughter has felt so abandoned that she has threatened to take her own life. But I'm extremely happy to know that at least I can live this part of my life and give my children love.

I used to be tormented by powerful nightmares. All of us constantly dreamt about Dad and various horrible things he did. The pain. The terror. His disgusting groans... the smell... the hands... the hard, cold look in his eyes. I used to wake up shaking as I lay there in bed, feeling as if it was actually happening, over and over again. I couldn't cope with my anxiety and had to take medication.

In the therapy, I get help picking out my memories, one piece at a time. At first I don't want to, and protest angrily. TT encourages me to try, just for a minute. I lose the sense of time and space. One minute feels like several hours. Everything's happening again — all the assaults, all the pain and terror inflicted on me. The wounds are deep. My anxiety wells up with full strength. My heart pounds, my body feels paralysed and I feel as if I'm going to die. In the nightmares, I'm alone and helpless. But in the sessions with TT, I confront that anxiety in safety. She holds my hand while I struggle. I feel the warmth. I'm safe, and the shame lets go of me. I'm not the one who's disgusting — I'm not the one who's done wrong!

I hear TT's soothing voice: *'It happened THEN, not NOW.'* Over and over again, she says it. And urges me to look around: *'What do you hear? Do you hear my voice? Where are you now?'* She's there with me. I feel her hand and it helps me discover that I'm not there, but here. Daring to trust her — that she'll stay and not abandon me — takes a long time. Now my confidence in her is strong. Otherwise, I'd never have had the strength to face the fear that rushed around inside me, in my various personality parts.

Jigsaw pieces falling into place

Letting hard stuff come out is painful during the seconds it takes and the minute after. But it's worth it. Afterwards, I experience indescribable relief. What's happened is impossible to forget: all that's been was broken and torn in me, the terror and chaos, the electric shocks and pills... But now all the jigsaw pieces have finally ended up in the right place. Now I grasp why I've felt so disgusting, and know who the crazy one was. As a child, you don't understand that.

Between therapy sessions, I can listen to TT's voice, which she's recorded for me. *'It happened THEN, not NOW. It's over.'* It really helps when the anxiety comes back. With her voice as support, I can calm myself.

Before the therapy, I experienced the violence inside me every day. Now, after a few years of therapy, the abuses belong to the past. My mental problems, which no one was able to understand, have become intelligible. With understanding comes the opportunity to heal. I no longer have a single nightmare. If it starts happening I think, *Okay, it's a dream; he can no longer hurt me. I'm here now, in this reality.* I know the way back to myself.

Love

It's impossible to describe how *angry* I sometimes used to be. The rage was so strong. I could really *hate*. Tana quarrelled with the doctors and my husband. The staff didn't understand what the anger was about, couldn't handle it and instead argued back — so it just got worse.

One moment I was a very sweet girl, the next I was mean. Tana could stay angry for a very long time. Sometimes it took several days for her to calm down. It wasn't easy for my husband to cope with my mood swings. Tana wanted to push through a divorce. When I ask my husband how he put up with me, he just looks at me and says, *'Love.'* I still have moods, but now I'm just angry for a while, and it's about something that's actually happened here and now, not old rubbish from the past. The rage, frustration and hatred that I thought were me have released their grip on me.

Looking back on my life, I wonder how I actually coped with living. It feels like I was someone else. Today, I can see that my survival was thanks to Tana, in a way. She fought for life, and gave me strength. The nice one wouldn't have had the strength to live.

Everyday joy

Now I want to make my own decisions. But I don't want a divorce. Being able to decide for myself is wonderful — I haven't been allowed to do that earlier in my life. Before, my husband had *several* parts of my personality to deal with; now there's just *one* Yasmine. I know he's put up with it because he loves me. Now he counts on me being well and dares to build a future with me.

Magnus, the kids and I have a cosy time at home. In the evening, we have supper together and talk about what happened during the day. We laugh a lot together. We joke and tease one another. I can threaten them, saying, *'If you don't do as I say now, I'll go mad and end up in hospital.'* Then Magnus and the children answer, *'Oh, when are you going?'* or *'We'll give you a lift there straightaway!'* And then we all laugh. It feels great.

My eldest girl's grown up now. She didn't have an easy time, because I couldn't take care of her. Now she comes here to visit. We bake together and enjoy ourselves. There's a lot of closeness between us. It feels like I've got my daughter back. She understands.

A secure life

If I'd never met TT, my children would have no mother today. I don't think I would have survived without therapy, or they would have had to visit me in a closed unit. I don't want to think about what might have happened. I'm just extremely grateful that I finally got the right help.

It's taken time to find my way home. The journey's been long. Before, everything felt threatening and dangerous. Now I think the world's beautiful. I've left the past behind me. I never, ever, think of suicide any more. I'm so thankful. My in-laws love me just as I am — as their own child. We have full confidence in one another, although I've been so ill.

Of course I can still be sad, like everyone else. But I'm no longer unable to stop shaking from anxiety, nor am I alone in the dark any more. I'm living a secure life. Magnus has really proved to be a good husband that I can trust. For several years when I was ill, I didn't let him sleep in our bed. I couldn't cope with any closeness. It's hard to understand how he managed, but he just says that we're married, and he'd promised to love me for better or for worse. Living with a man who protects me has been absolutely crucial. Now that I'm well, I like being close to him. At last I'm free to love without being scared. My husband has got me back. Now he gets my love. A new world's opening up.

Dream of Thailand

There's been so much grief in my family in Thailand. So many suicides. In my old homeland, all the relatives are so close. The family feeling remains, although I've never seen them. We've had four funerals in a short time. My sister died of cancer. Two weeks later, our mother died. My sister had four children aged from 3 to 13. Her husband couldn't cope with looking after them. He hanged himself. The 13-year-old was raped by four guys. People gossiped, and she got no support. Now she's hanged herself too. The children model themselves on what they see. They learn that suicide's the only solution to despair. I get sad, but can handle my feelings.

Sometimes I dream of going back. I long for the food, the scents and the people. But no one's left there now. So many are dead. In the dream, I want to travel back home to Sweden, but I can't buy a ticket for the flight. I'm stuck. The dream becomes a nightmare. No, I won't go to Thailand.

I love my life. My husband, children and job. And I've learnt to set limits and say no, without being unkind. I'm an adult woman who dares to show who I am. I say what I think; I laugh when I'm happy and cry when I get sad. There's room for every feeling in me. Sometimes I have to struggle with painful things but I'm still secure. Yesterday I felt a pang of envy of my teenage daughter because she has a loving father that she can be close to without having to be afraid. I never got to experience that, and it makes me sad. Then, a moment later, comes gratitude that my children can feel the love from their father.

Joy of life

The older people I work with appreciate me and how lively, and full of cheer and energy, I am. They help me feel valuable. I really enjoy talking to them. We have a good laugh together. They may look old on the outside, but their zest for life still burns inside. I get masses of love from them.

In the end, we'll all die. It doesn't matter which day is my turn. I want to live NOW. Laughing, joking. So much feels fun. Having a job is wonderful. If I'm free for a few days, I usually go there and join them for coffee. My colleagues are so kind. They take me as I am.

I'm truly happy, right here in my heart. I appreciate life. That's no pretence. Everything's genuine. I've cried enough in my life. That's over now. Nothing can stop me.

Whole at last

Yes, it does feel like I lost my childhood. I never got to be the little one. But I'm not ashamed of what happened. It wasn't my fault. I was a small, vulnerable child. Responsibility rests on the adults who abused me. In the therapy, I found the little child in me and lovingly took care of her.

CHAPTER 11

A function for every dissociative part

This book's stories about life with dissociation show how several different parts of the personality can arise in a person who is exposed to trauma early in life. The small child's fragmented world does not fuse together as the child grows up and, as a result, no unified personality ever develops. The various parts may be said to be frozen in the past, living on in the perception of threats.

Every part of the personality has its own identity, with its own abilities, memories and feelings. But who, in fact, are the different parts? What characterises them? What strategies do they each use in their quest for security? How does the body act when a particular part takes command? How does the dissociative part perceive the body? Where in the body are memories primarily located?

Everyday part of the personality — ANP

The 'ordinary', seemingly well-functioning part of the personality is usually termed 'ANP', which stands for 'apparently normal part of the personality'. One and the same person can develop several ANPs.

For the sake of simplicity, we choose to call ANP the 'everyday part of the personality'. This part puts all its strength and energy into being a manager in daily life. It decides when the person sleeps, eats, drinks, goes to the bathroom and is active and social. ANP runs the person's everyday life and strives to make everything work optimally. This part works hard to avoid traumatic memories and carries a heavy burden.

If the person's external life rolls on without disturbance, this may be quite workable, but ANP usually has difficulty when an event triggers memories of previous worrying or threatening experiences. To make life manageable, the everyday part of the personality systematically tries to avoid such situations. ANP may be said to suffer from phobia when it seeks at all costs to avoid feelings, closeness and much more. As long as the strategy of avoiding everything painful and frightening is working, the everyday part of the personality can maintain control.

Survival part of the personality — EP

One or more 'emotional parts' (EPs) of the personality, which are highly sensitive to stress, accompany ANP (or ANPs). Here, we choose to call them 'survival parts of the personality' or EPs. These dissociative parts are always based on the need to protect themselves. Through various behaviours, they try to escape the experiences and memories of what has happened.

The survival parts of the personality carry strong feelings linked to their painful memories. They all want to protect themselves, but usually have completely different solutions to how this should happen. Some parts of an emotional nature adopt a very strongly controlling position ('EP-C Control'). This part's behavioural pattern is strongly linked to becoming active in situations in which it perceives a need for control. Its vulnerability is hidden away. Anger often helps this part of the personality to take control, and not infrequently this part has a phobia of someone getting close. Then it fights for its life.

At the same time, other survival parts of the personality often take a completely different role, as vulnerable victims ('EP-Fragility'). This is an emotional part in which vulnerability is in the fore. This part is usually quick to take flight, but may simultaneously have a strong need to seek protection in a relationship with a caring person. This may involve a desperate desire for attachment. Its attachment-related crying — the crying we are born with, aimed at eliciting care from our caregivers — may be loud. The struggle to avoid separation may overshadow everything. Often, these parts have perceived their only chance of survival as being through obedience and submission.

Examples of survival parts of the personality

A dissociative part of the personality may do everything possible to defend itself from closeness. It does so by not letting anyone near, because of phobic avoidance behaviour in this part's relationships with others. This survival part of the personality is terrified of attachment and, when it comes to getting close to others, often ruins everything and acts destructively.

There may be one or more survival parts of the personality that mimic the perpetrator (or perpetrators) in their attitude. Such a part can appear very tough. The defence action system is strongly dominant in these EPs. In their inner dynamics, such parts often have a terrifying influence on the other parts, including the everyday one. The survival part of the personality that mimics the perpetrator rarely sees any other option than to try to seize control itself, and behaves accordingly. Vulnerability feels perilous, and it shies away from closeness.

There may be an extremely severe internal struggle among different parts in one and the same person. They want different things and have different strategies when they feel insecure. They must do things their own way, save themselves or fight for them all. These EPs are utterly confused in chronological terms. They live in the past, often in trying times of great trauma, and continue to defend themselves as if the dangerous incidents were happening now. They often misinterpret current events. Their behaviour, as seen by others, may be extremely bizarre, since they often have powerful flashbacks and perceive the traumatising events as occurring in the present.

Several everyday parts of the personality

Several everyday parts of the personality may form in one person. One of them may have studied; this may be the part that goes to work and is an accomplished professional. Another everyday part is dominant and takes charge of family life, the children and what life demands. The everyday parts of the personality often have different main tasks and have originated in various periods of the patient's life. If so, what we call 'dissociative identity disorder' (DID) is involved.

DID is the most severe dissociative diagnosis. Patients are often unaware of their many identities. Trust is non-existent. The person presents multiple symptoms — usually a combination of dissociative, affective, post-traumatic and physical — such as memory gaps, hallucinations and inexplicable, destructive behaviour. The multifaceted symptoms of DID make it hard to detect that a person is suffering from this disorder.

Splitting varies in depth

Each part of the personality has its own characteristics and serves its own purpose for our survival. One may be responsible for bodily care, ensuring that the person gets food to eat and so on. Another part ensures that the children are looked after properly, while a third protects physical integrity when there is a real or perceived threat. Each part of the personality carries out one or more tasks and perseveres in achieving its goal. All the parts belong to a common system, but none of them governs overall. There is no inner agent that harmonises them as a conductor unifies a choir's vocal parts.

Understanding how deeply divided the various parts of the personality are from one another becomes one of the therapist's basic tasks. Exploring which parts may know of and perhaps get support from one another, and which are at loggerheads, pulling in different directions, is another need. What is their internal interaction like? Who is shouting, screaming and scaring the others? Is there any conscious interaction and collaboration among the parts? Which parts know about the existence of which, and in that case how do they see one another? How do they interrelate when one part chooses to be entirely dominant? What is their communication like? How well do they separate one another's various roles and deficiencies? The list of questions that need answers is long.

The various parts' depth and degree of their separation from one another may vary. Sometimes, some information and feelings seep from one part to another. There are times when the parts toss remembered images and experiences from one to another. At other times they do not communicate at all, like islands, largely cut off from one another. Sometimes, dissociated people are unaware of their alternative identities. Parts of the personality may be very careful to keep their own existence, and their stories, secret from one another.

Flashbacks

The survival parts of a person with trauma-related dissociation may penetrate the seemingly well-functioning portion of the personality, with a variable and sometimes powerful impact on the person's life. On the other hand, the survival parts of the personality can be kept at a distance for a long time and not allowed to break into the everyday part's existence. During this time, the person may be able to work hard, study intensively or run some other life-filling project. Building a family may be just this kind of commitment.

Then, suddenly, something may happen in life that prevents an almost total avoidance of the person's story. The EPs' egos push their way to the fore. These emotionally charged parts may be more or less independent. They may be aware of one another to some extent or not at all. They may simply be unaware, or have just begun to get an inkling, that other parts of the person exist. From time to time, EPs may take over ANPs' entire behaviour and sphere of experience. They can also lead parallel lives, thrusting themselves forward on various occasions, often with anxiety or strong memories.

As if the danger were present now

The emotionally dominated survival parts of the personality often get flashbacks. Recollections pour in. The parts are chronologically confused and remain, more or less constantly, in the perilous period when their trauma took place. If they turn their attention inward, into themselves, their inner world is full of triggers. Each part can have feelings, strong bodily sensations or thoughts that activate anxiety and make them perceive the old incidents as recurring now. Other parts, by whispering to or shouting at another, may spark off the latter's anxiety, fear or anxiety.

When the more emotionally charged parts are suppressed, the everyday part of the personality may perceive itself as unemotional, dulled, robotic, cut off from the body, or severely stressed and beset with perceptions of the world's strangeness.

Everyday life

Another passenger on the Metro starting to hold forth at a high volume may, for a dissociative person, result in activation of the various parts of the personality. They begin arguing among themselves about how to deal with the situation and find a secure refuge. The inner person becomes chaotic.

Every EP has its own solution to the situation, depending on how these parts assess it and which approach or measures they themselves have developed most. One who wishes to escape wants to get off the train. Another who feels like fighting wants to meddle and argue with the other passengers. One part may become terrified and completely blocked. Wishing only to become invisible, it may prompt the person to crawl down behind a fellow passenger. Another part thinks the argument is her own fault. If she hadn't been sitting there, or looking at him, this would never have happened. Like an insecure small child who believes her actions rule the world, she must be sure to 'do the right thing'; otherwise, dangerous things happen. One part just wants to sit close, hold hands or be embraced, and has a constant longing for security.

The most severe results

When the splitting is deepest, the parts have well-constructed, fully-fledged psychobiological phenomena, known as action systems. These are self-organising and self-stabilising. Measurably differing blood pressure for 'individuals' in the system may then sometimes be found. One part of the personality may be completely blind, another seeing. One may be right-handed, another left-handed. They often have completely different handwriting. Sometimes they speak different languages. The parts have genuinely grown up as 'individuals' in their own right that, when they appear and take over, have their physical and mental starting point in their perception of the 'self'.

Thus, there are several subsystems in one and the same body that may say, *'I want...'* or *'I am...'* More than one individual cannot, of course, coexist in the same body, but their conviction is so strong that it gives a complete perceived 'self' to every part of the personality that dominates the body at one time or another.

However, information often seeps from one part to another, especially when therapeutic work on the system begins. Then, the parts' conviction of their own independence is gradually eroded.

It is a long, intensive task. By the time the dissociative parts begin to understand that they share the same body, which cannot be hurt or killed without them all being affected, they have taken a major step towards recovery.

During the journey to a healthy life, there is much to work through: what is going on in the present, as well as what happened in the past; bodily experiences; relationships among the parts of the personality; and so on. The goal — for the traumatised to get over the suffering caused by being so fragmented and haunted by previous events — makes the work highly meaningful. When they can eventually integrate their dissociative parts into individuals who are subject to a single captain and sail under the same flag, it becomes possible to live without being constantly thwarted by demons from the past.

Second chance in life

Dissociative syndrome as a result of traumatisation is, as we have seen, a very severe and complicated disorder. Is getting well even feasible? The answer is YES. Healing and recovery often take a long time, but are entirely possible, just as the interviewees' narratives show.

Work in the treatment room reveals high-level group dynamics. The patient's whole system, with all the different parts of the personality, must be invited. Addressing the seemingly well-functioning ANP is not enough. Inside the patient, full-scale armed hostilities may be under way. Some parts may be utterly terrified of another, a sharpshooter whose ammunition is harsh words, accusations, threats and condemnations.

Gathering all the parts of the personality that fight, oppress one another or hide is a tough challenge. The process can be extremely frustrating for the various parts. But *everyone* must be on board. Slowly, with awareness through every sense and with responsiveness and compassion, a trusting alliance is built, sometimes first with every part of the personality separately and gradually also among them all.

The healing presupposes that you manage to create so much balance and trust that all the parts can bear to go through painful memories, and dare to approach one another, change their relationships and, step by step, integrate to become a whole, connected person.

Soon we shall look more closely at the requirements of successful treatment. Being a survivor who gets the right help and can then live a balanced and healthy life is, as a severely traumatised person described it, *'a second chance in life, so totally different from the first phase — a laugh full of happiness that never really disappears.'*

First, however, we need to clear up some misunderstandings around diagnoses that are sometimes mixed up.

Confused terms: schizophrenia, MPD and DID

The hope is that what you have read so far in this book has brought some clarity to the phenomenon of trauma-related dissociation. You may be wondering what the difference between dissociation and schizophrenia really is. Dr Jekyll and Mr Hyde were, surely, two completely different people in one and the same body — so he was probably schizophrenic, wasn't he? And on television, documentaries about people with multiple personality disorder are shown... So which is which?

Trauma-related dissociation is, as you have seen, a very complex area. Our aim is to make it as easy as possible to understand. In this book, we cannot go into detail about what distinguishes DID from other diagnoses. All the same, we want to list some words that, we hope, can shed light on the often confused terminology.

'Dissociative Identity Disorder' (DID) is a modern term. 'Multiple Personality Disorder' (MPD) was used until 1994 for virtually the same psychiatric condition, in which the patient has multiple personality parts. But that was many years ago, and much more is now known. The diagnostic system has changed. The previous criteria for diagnosing MPD differed from those applied today for diagnosing DID. Another important change is that DID is now no longer categorised as a personality disorder, but as a stress-related mental disorder instead.

The concept of multiple personality disorder appeared in 1980, in the internationally recognised medical publication *Diagnostic and Statistical Manual of Mental Disorders* (DSM). One reason why the name was later changed was a wish to remove the 'Hollywood stamp' associated with the diagnosis after films like *Dr Jekyll and Mr Hyde*, *The Three Faces of Eve* and *Sybil*. Back in 1886, in his novella about Dr Jekyll and Mr Hyde, the author Robert Louis Stevenson described two completely different identities in one and the same person. This book and these films do not, of course, present DID, MPD or schizophrenia in a knowledgeable, objective way: rather, they reflect contemporary fantasies about the phenomena.

Psychotic or not?

Sometimes, the term schizophrenic is used for characters with 'split personality' that films with a popular appeal have attempted to portray. In *Me, Myself & Irene*, Jim Carrey plays a 'schizophrenic' man with two different personality parts. Perhaps one of the first known mix-ups is found in a text written by the poet T. S. Eliot back in 1933. The misleading use of the word 'schizophrenia' to convey the sense of a 'split psyche' has evidently contributed to the terminological confusion.

It is therefore very important to grasp that DID and schizophrenia are not the same but, on the contrary, two different types of mental disorder. Schizophrenia is a severe psychiatric illness belonging to the category of psychotic illnesses. The perception of being persecuted often predominates. Delusions and hallucinations are common symptoms.

However, schizophrenic patients do not display multiple, distinctly different parts of the personality.

Nevertheless, patients with DID and schizophrenia may sometimes present with similar symptoms and this, of course, impedes understanding. To observers, people with DID may initially seem psychotic although they are not. A further complication is that a person with DID *can* become psychotic. One dissociative part of the personality in someone with DID *can* actually become psychotic on occasion without thereby being schizophrenic. In other words, the truth is by no means simple.

CHAPTER 12

Using compassion, self-compassion and mindfulness

This chapter contains ideas, knowledge and experience relating to treatment of PTSD and trauma-related dissociation. The intention is to understand vulnerable and severely suffering people better, and help them improve their lives. The more of us in caring professions there are who are keen to learn more, so as to help severely traumatised people, the better.

If you, the reader, are personally affected we hope you find here, in this chapter, some advice on how to get the right treatment. You should not hesitate to ask for what you think you need.

The crucial meeting

The prospects of successful treatment are enhanced by the patient and therapist meeting as equals — at least, on the most equal footing attainable. Clearly, the therapist possesses theoretical knowledge and has long gathered experience from meeting others who, after striving to get well, have done so. Nevertheless, patients are experts on their own life story and problems. They know what they have been through and are experiencing now, and what their suffering and inner world are like. Together, the patient and therapist form a team. Joining forces enables them, step by step, to reach their common goal: making life as harmonious and healthy as possible for the trauma survivor.

A trusting rapport between patient and therapist is crucial for effective treatment. Trust emerges gradually and, as we have seen, requires continuity. We therapists must remember that survivors often forget information we give them. We must then provide it again; but sometimes this may be easy to overlook. If the therapist is suddenly replaced and the secure relationship interrupted, it may greatly damage the patient. Sadly, this happens all too often in the care sector today. The sense of security that comes from meeting the same therapist over a long period cannot be emphasised enough.

We describe complex conditions that are very difficult to treat. This book depicts total confusion and terror, and the personal stories bear witness to indescribable suffering. At the same time, these narratives show how traumatised people can achieve greater understanding of themselves and, step by step, find their way to well-being.

The echo of childhood is strong, but change is possible. The deep wounds heal slowly. An avoidant, ambivalent or disorganised attachment is replaced by a newly acquired, secure one. By being in a trusting relationship with the therapist while practising mindfulness, compassion and self-compassion, patients themselves boost recovery in the central nervous system. As one of the patients put it, *'I can understand both myself and reality now. It's wonderful that I can feel this secure!'*

Aware with the senses

PTSD affects the *whole* person. When reactions to trauma have not healed naturally but, instead, resulted in a life marred by post-traumatic symptoms, focused work is needed. What is known as simple PTSD is a condition that a person can overcome with relative ease, after one or a few treatments. This does not mean that victims do not suffer — they often suffer a great deal — but that simple PTSD is not hard to treat. For more severe dissociative conditions, on the other hand, longer treatments are required.

Many people living with trauma-related dissociation have found their experience of the care services very unhelpful. Their suffering from painful events early in their lives has continued. Their self-compassion is non-existent. They have often had several previous diagnoses, and their many years of therapy have not led to any major progress. Memory gaps are also common. Typically, these patients behave very differently in the treatment room from one occasion to the next. Their rapid changes of appearance, voice and mood somewhat confuse the therapist. We therapists must listen with humility when the patient shows the way.

Providing psychotherapy challenges therapists' ability to be securely mindful here and now, responsive and compassionate at every new moment. They need to show their compassion and a genuine desire to relieve their patients' burdens, not with distance and an intellectualising attitude but by giving them respectful space. This is indeed a tough challenge. People with structural dissociation have a history of relational trauma. They therefore have numerous antennae out, sensing every nuance and picking up on unspoken messages as few others can do.

Patients do not tell their stories with words alone. To take note of subtle signals, we therapists must work to be mindful with all our senses. We must constantly remind ourselves to listen and pay attention to what is being said between the lines. This unspoken communication is at least as important as the words used. Much is conveyed through small shifts in facial expression, body language or actions that may initially be hard to understand. Often, not even the patients are aware of what they are relating.

Therapists need to know what to look for, be open to surprises and detect the most unexpected manifestations of trauma and dissociation. At almost every meeting, we learn something new. None of us, of course, can be mindful and observant all the time. We can all only strive to be so.

Identifying the problems

Self-assessment scales provide clues as to how severely traumatised patients are, the trauma level they are located on and their degree of dissociation. There may even be a structural dissociation.

Through interviews, various symptoms are surveyed. These sessions need to identify traumatic experiences to some extent. What has happened in this person's life to leave its mark? Have the incidents been isolated or recurrent? How did these experiences affect the various dissociative parts of the patient's personality and their thoughts, feelings and behaviour? What do they think of themselves? What do they think of others? What supportive people have been and are now there for them? What are the patient's relationships and daily life like now? What beliefs and generalisations are typical of the patient's various personality parts? Assessment interviews need to clarify this and much more before the treatment starts.

The path to successful treatment

Efforts to help anyone recover from severe traumatisation and trauma-related dissociation can be truly rewarding. For the victim, the focused treatment work can provide completely new scope for a rich, meaningful life. But there is no shortcut. People who were traumatised early in life must work very hard to leave their past experience behind. Dedicated work is necessary. No external event can loosen the brakes and get life to roll happily along by itself.

If you, the reader, are a trauma survivor, look not only at what we write about the lack of shortcuts or the need for hard work. Read the lines about the potential that exists for a rich, meaningful and healthy life if you get the right help. Read these words, so full of hope, repeatedly. Otherwise, the brain focuses automatically on negative thoughts that crop up, and you risk running out of steam.

'It happened to me, but that was then'

For people suffering from trauma-related dissociation, it is difficult at all levels to realise that

- the traumatising experience really happened
- it happened to me in particular
- the mental and behavioural actions that take place are mine (*I'm the one doing this*)
- the threatening events are over, and happened a long time ago
- the self in the past is the same self as in the present
- an intact, integrated perception of myself as *one* self, physically here in the present, is lacking.

Trauma-related dissociation is simply a lack of integration. The person is not fully convinced, cognitively and emotionally, by the thought that *it happened to me, but it happened then.*

The task of connecting one's life experiences and achieving a unified perception of oneself — *I'm me; I have a past and a future* — has stopped short. The capacity to perceive oneself as a person in a context is lacking. Working step by step to attain these insights is a time-consuming, but tremendously meaningful process.

One of TT's patients was delighted when she began to understand that, as she put it, '*This whole spectrum of impressions is mine, and they belong to a context. It's wonderful — I had no idea.*'

FIFTH STORY

By the time Joanna meets TT, she has been unable to work for ten long years despite her academic degree. *'In the past decade, life has just been heavy, black grief and total confusion, which I don't remember much about,'* she says at the beginning of the therapy.

In the past she has worked hard, studying and initially working in her new role as a professional. Not managing to make use of her knowledge distresses her. For as long as she can, Joanna has done her utmost, but she is eventually unable to fend off the repercussions of her upbringing any longer.

No more can she fully let herself go, impelled by her inner driving force of learning and work. No longer is she able to perform well, and she takes sick leave. Physical pain stops her training as a runner, although her passion for sport has previously been another life-sustaining force.

Joanna is referred to TT. A skilled young psychiatrist has finally understood something important, and ensures that a wise person in charge of psychiatric services decides that Joanna should be referred for trauma therapy until she completes it. Today, thanks to this well-advised initiative, Joanna is the healthy mother of a lovely little one-year-old daughter.

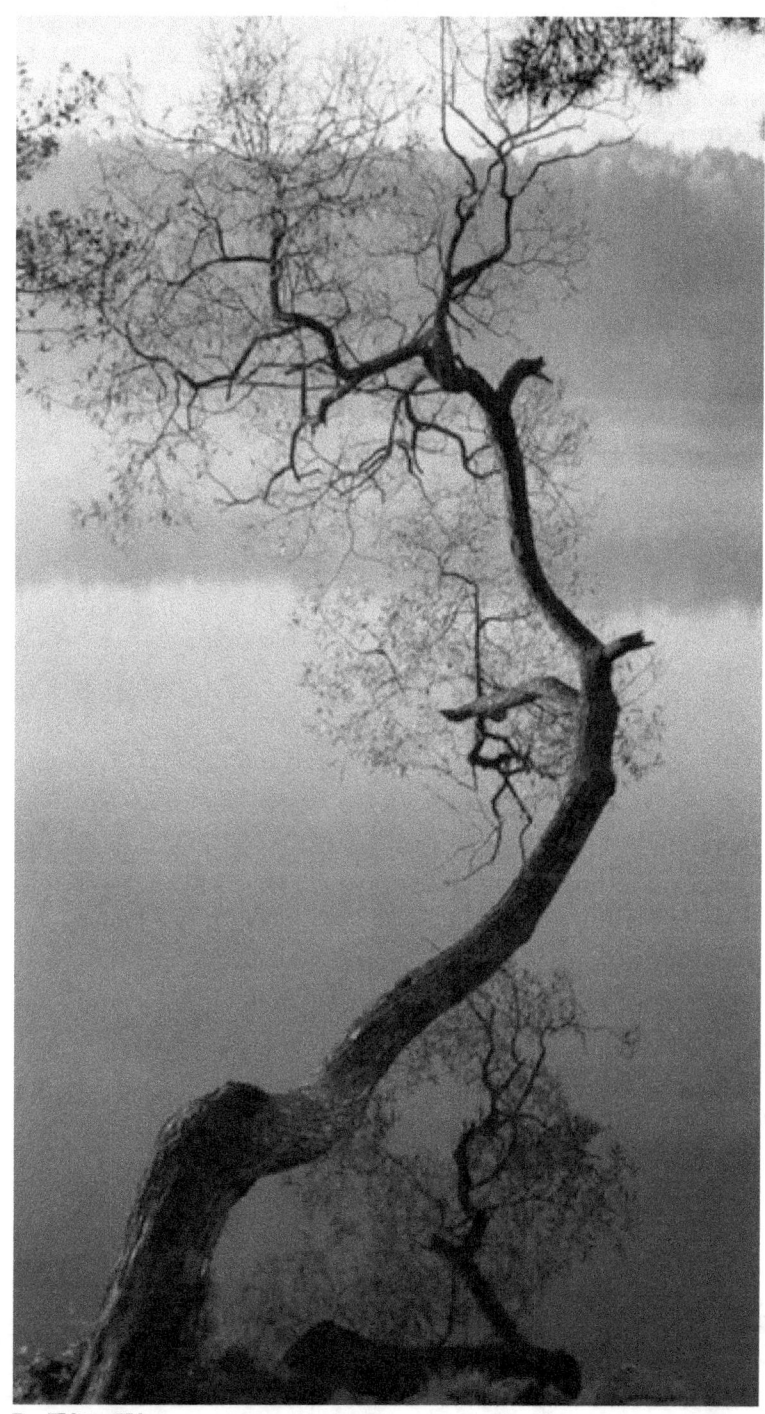

By Elina Ehn

Joanna

Joanna's father exploits her sexually. The incomprehensible acts keep happening, over and over again. He takes his daughter with him to other adults who abuse her. Repeatedly, she is severely assaulted.

To protect herself, she flees from reality. In her powerless state, various parts of her personality have to bear the pain and terror. Joanna lives in an inner chaos with 16 different parts, each one pulling in its own direction.

'Throughout my childhood, I suffer gross sexual exploitation. There's no escape. It's like disappearing into a black hole. Reliving and working through those terrifying memories and not having to bear them alone really make a difference. My whole life is changed. For the first time, the memories are going back into the past, and I no longer suffer from nightmares.

'Now I realise all those troubles are over. We can look through the same eyes, breathe at the same time and smile at the same things. We know we're safe. Before, not all my parts knew that. Each was isolated, as if on an island. Now I walk around as a single, whole person on a solid continent.'

I've always been shy and quiet, and felt scared and exposed. Going to day nursery didn't work. Every time Mum left me there, I was terribly upset.

Mum had to be at home with us and she worked as a childminder. So I had other children to play with, which I quite enjoyed. That was when I was really small and we lived in Halland, in the south of Sweden.

After our move to the city of Västerås, life becomes harder. I am very shy and feel different. Staying in the background both at school and at home, I make myself invisible.

Some girls at school are really nasty. To protect myself, I try to read from their behaviour what's about to happen and adapt myself. I'm afraid, just as I am at home. The world feels dangerous.

All my own fault

My upbringing is characterised by obeying Dad and constantly thinking about not making Mum sad. She's so sensitive. We all often feel sorry for Mum. I have to take responsibility for her well-being. If I don't do what she wants, she kind of disappears — retreats into herself and punishes me with her absence.

To some extent, the demand for adaptation is unspoken. No words are needed. I take in the body language, looks and energies, and the silence speaks volumes. But sometimes Dad says very clearly that it's my fault when Mum's unhappy. He says things like, *'That was unnecessary, Joanna. Look, now Mum got sad. And it's your fault.'* Then I feel ashamed, wrong and useless. I have no adult to turn to and am left alone with the blame. I learn to put my own needs and wishes aside.

When I'm eight, my little sister is born. I feel great responsibility for the little one. I take on a lot and sacrifice myself. Why? First, I have to make things easier for Mum. Second, I want to protect my sister. I feel it very strongly, my responsibility to protect her. And I want to do the right thing, too. That's my only way of getting affirmation: being praised when I do something good.

Alone with the guilt

Early on, I learn two unspoken rules. First, in our family we mustn't feel anything — at least not me. Second, in our family we mustn't talk about anything that upsets my parents.

I'm brought up to shut out everything unpleasant I experience. It's a matter of shoving the nasty stuff down, way down, inside me — denying its existence.

I become good at pushing the shutdown button, but pay a high price.

All the same, I'm totally abandoned. Left in the terror. Alone in shame and then guilt. In my thoughts, I often beat myself up. I accuse myself: *It's all my own fault and I should have done things differently.*

I work hard to keep the terror and the guilt at bay. But my body remembers. So I have to live with a lot of tension and, later, fibromyalgia. The pain has to go somewhere. My body stores all these troublesome feelings and painful memories.

Just groping at first, then...

In my earliest conscious memories, I'm three or four years old. Little Joanna is walking by Dad's side, holding his hand. I feel happy to be with him — my little hand in his big one. I have a strong wish to share something nice. To sit on his lap, be held and hugged. My Dad and me. But he starts coming to my bed in the evenings and touching me.

One day, he leads me down into the basement of our house. It's cold. *What are we going to do down here?* Then something terrible happens that I don't understand at all. Dad starts feeling my body. To start with it's playful, but the fun quickly turns into something horrid. He crosses every boundary and I get really scared and confused.

Dad coaxes me to touch him and tricks me into letting him touch me. My body reacts. There are two extremes. For a brief second it's nice when he touches me. He isn't rough and his voice is kind when he whispers, *'You see how nice it is.'* But soon it slips into pain. I'm terribly scared and don't understand at all what's happening. Everything feels confusing, unpleasant and shameful. Dad's there, but still I'm completely alone — in a turmoil of shock and horror.

Afterwards, Dad says I'm lovely, so lovely, and I'm his girl. I don't want to be lovely if it means I have to be involved in that. But I don't dare say so.

There must be something wrong with me, not liking what Dad does. He says it's something fine and good we have together. I love his kind voice saying that, but my body protests. I don't understand a thing. I can't trust either Dad or myself. *It must be my fault!* The scared — in fact, terrified and confused — little me and the sad little me face an impossible task: to carry all that inside.

Big black hole

The unfathomable abuse happens again and again. Little Joanna walks there by Dad's side, holding his hand. He leads me down to the basement. How I long to be close to him! But not for this kind of closeness, not at all. The terror of what's going to happen makes me sort of leave my body.

I know what to expect. Down there in the cold basement, he assaults and hurts me. Terror and pain. I'm totally alone. There's no one I can turn to, nobody to protect or hold me, to stand up against the menace. Dad films what he's doing to me. There are no limits.

I shut myself off to stop feeling all the nastiness. My body's there, but I'm not. It's like disappearing into a big, black hole. Everything's cold and naked around me. It's like seeing myself from the outside. There my body lies. *Supposing I die?* I don't dare struggle against it, thinking perhaps I'll die if I do.

Although I don't understand what was happening, I feel the shame afterwards. I'm so much at the mercy of Dad's incomprehensible acts. I can't tell anyone what he does. Talking to Mum would be unthinkable. I can well imagine how sad she'd be. She'd be unable to cope with it. Dad threatens me, saying Mum will disappear if I reveal what's going on. He makes me feel that Mum's survival is my responsibility. He deceives me into thinking it's my job in life to make sure Mum doesn't go under.

I know no one else either that I dare turn to. So I keep quiet and try to understand how I should behave to escape from it all.

Turning to ice

A good little girl in me makes sure I'm nice and obedient. Superficially, she's cheerful and happy, just as I'm expected to be. That part of me can be seen. Mum has no understanding of all that's hidden beneath the surface. Looking back now, I think it's incredible that it's possible to live like that. But it worked.

At home, I always have to be on my guard. I need to keep a lookout all the time. Dad may come at any time and take me to different places. I can never feel safe. I'm a bundle of nerves, with tension running deep into my body. It's like walking on a minefield and trying to figure out where to tread, how I have to move so as not to put a foot wrong. I don't know what I'm doing to provoke his desire to begin doing those vile things.

I remember sitting and drawing, completely in my fantasy world. For a short while, I forget the threat that constantly hangs over me. Suddenly Dad's there, giving me that look. The terror I feel at that moment is hard to describe. I want to run away. Panic rushes through me, but I become totally rigid. I turn to ice. What's going to happen? Dad rules. I obey. And I know there must be something wrong with me. But what do I have to be like to get out of it?

Some part of me looks up to Dad and absorbs his contemptuous attitude towards me. Eventually, I understand that this is a male–female thing, and feel I'd very much like to be a boy. Might I be able to get away then?

That look...

When the outings to the basement begin, Dad uses playfulness to get what he wants — for a while. Then, instead, he uses the assaults as a punishment. Coldly, he says I've been disobedient and have myself to blame. The terrible stuff I'm subjected to is my own fault. Now he says it straight out: that he has to rape me because I'm so awful.

The result is that I work even harder to oblige him. I make the greatest possible effort to avoid doing anything wrong. But it's hard to avoid doing whatever makes him switch from my usual Dad to the strange Dad. I don't know what it is.

Forgetting to be vigilant, for a single moment, can be terribly dangerous. I remember us having dinner together, the whole family. I don't remember what we're talking about, but we're having quite a nice time together around the dining table. At that moment, I relax. Suddenly I look in Dad's direction and see his eyes. That look! Everything shatters. The joy, the security and the sense of being an ordinary family are swept away in that second. I know what lies ahead — but not how to get away.

If I try to slip away, he'll get angry and hold me hard. I know that trying to protect myself will be punished. So when the time comes, after dinner, it's best to keep as calm as possible. Go with him. Endure.

Male strangers

Sometimes Dad says he rapes me because I'm so pretty and lovely, at other times because I have to be punished. Sometimes he forces himself on me for no reason at all. I don't understand.

When I'm about five, Dad lets one of his friends come down to the basement with us. He lets him do the same horrible things to me. Why does Dad do that? It's incomprehensible.

The film camera reappears. Dad and the other man take turns raping me and filming each other's assaults. *'If you tell anyone about this, no one will believe you,'* Dad tells me. I believe him.

Soon he starts taking me to other men — once to a man I recognise, but usually to total strangers. Sometimes a woman also joins in abusing me, but mostly it's adult men I'm forced to meet.

The assaults take place in various places: in the basement, where my father usually takes me, but also in unfamiliar flats, in the homes of male strangers. I particularly remember an apartment that's empty and seems to be used just for the abuse. Everything's prepared. There are ropes, knives, bottles and other weapons they use when they rape me.

Like an object

Dad lets other men and women rape me. Several adults on a little girl. I'm scared and defenceless. He, my parent, is supposed to protect me. Instead, he completely hands me over, and seems to enjoy being able to offer me to others to abuse. I'm dependent on him and can't understand how I should behave to avoid these terrifying experiences.

I carry powerful images, etched deep into my brain and body. Big people jeering at me, taking all my clothes off… I remember their voices, but not what they say. They touch my genitals. They get angry when I'm unwilling. Hold me down. I want to run out of there but am forced to be still. I can't move.

I become like an object to be tested. The men, in a party mood, urge one another on. It's as if each one is putting on a show for the others and they're competing to see who can cause me the most pain. At most, there are eight at a time. Eight adult male strangers. Inside me is nothing but chaos.

One moment, I'm told how pretty I am. Sexy. The next moment, the voices become hard. Contemptuous. They call me a whore and a cunt. *'You're going to die! You don't deserve to live. We'll finish you off. And you've got yourself to blame, you whore.'*

Away from the body

It's so awful, wanting to escape but being unable to get away. My whole body cries out for me to get out of there, but it's impossible. I'm completely stuck; my body just lies there and has to take it all, although it hurts so much.

It's all too much for me to stay there. All I can do is kind of shut down and leave my body mentally. I get away from what's going on, and freeze. Feel nothing — neither my body nor my pain. I disappear into another universe, and no longer have any contact with this world.

Inside me, everything comes to a standstill. Dad and the others don't notice anything. They're totally wrapped up in their own experience and don't grasp the fact that I've left my body.

After the rapes I don't know how they ended. I'm shut off. But Dad's pleased. I remember how he praises me, patting my head and saying what a lovely girl, what a good girl, I am. That ambivalent feeling that what he's done to me is horrible but that it still feels so pleasant to get the praise afterwards is very hard to take.

Then Dad pretends nothing has happened. It's so strange to me. One moment he's inflicting all that life-threatening nastiness on me, the next everything is as usual again. Perhaps, I think, those terrible things have to vanish from my consciousness for us to be able to live in the family.

Silence

It's hard to fully take it in that he, my father, can be so nasty. My terror is always present. I don't want to be seen or heard. I don't want attention. The lump stays in my throat, fixed there. I learn to be silent: otherwise, who knows what else may happen? I don't want to be in such pain, don't want to be stuck, unable to move, powerless. I don't want to... don't want it.

Over time, I begin to understand more about what's happening. Part of me knows it's all wrong: *life shouldn't be like this, it isn't okay*. But at the same time that's become normal for me — it has to be, somehow. Dad has always used me. I think it's the same for every girl, although it's never talked about. It's all I know.

When I realise, long afterwards, that life isn't like that for my friends, I feel totally filled with shame. I beat myself up, accusing myself of being weak and different. *Why can't I manage to be normal? What's wrong with me? Could I have done something differently so this would never happen? Why didn't I do it then? I'm to blame...* I go on and on thinking like that, with the thoughts going round and round in my head, and there's no way out. At the same time, the abuse goes on incessantly.

My dark secret

In the evenings, I lie in bed in the dark, with my torn genitals still hurting, and listen for Dad's steps in the hall. He may come at any time. Part of me needs to be constantly on guard. I never dare to relax. Lying there in bed, always in great suspense, is the source of all my tension.

The anxiety gnaws away at me. It applies to both myself and my little sister. Will he sneak into my room or go into hers? Whichever happens, it's terrible. I want to protect my little sister, but I can't. So I shut myself down...

Sometimes Dad comes in to me early in the morning. When he enters my room, it wakes me up. And I know what it means: the terror, the panic, like a thousand needles in the body. I just want to get out of there but I prepare myself, taking off my panties and spreading my legs. I know what's going to happen.

I'm so enormously ashamed but know there's no point arguing. Then it will just get worse. He'll get rough. Mean. Sadistic. I wish it could be over quickly — come to an end as fast as possible. Every tiny cell in my body gives up. I can't take it any more. I have no strength. That's my life; that's what it's like, and nothing can be done about it. I live in hell and just want to die. I can't bear to be there when it happens. I turn my face away, switch off and disappear.

Shut-down soul

Every morning, I feel bad. Abandoned. Even if Dad doesn't come that particular morning, waking up to a new day feels dangerous. The panic keeps flaring up. *How can I manage to go to school? How can I bear to go on living?*

Shutting myself down becomes my routine behaviour. In the end, a strong part of me is completely convinced that those dreadful things never happened. The parts of me that I later identify as the Denying One and the Everyday Girl go to school, put on a brave face and act normal. The Little Scared One and the Sad One are then completely switched off. All those parts of me don't know about one another's existence and never talk to one another.

In spite of everything, school is mostly fun. Maths and physical education are my favourite subjects. But I find it hard to relax. Sometimes, for a while, I can laugh and have fun with the other children, but usually my shyness and feeling of outsiderness are in the way. The Little One is too scared and sad to join in and play. She has gone into hiding and is cowering somewhere deep inside me where no one can see her.

The feeling of being a bad person grows stronger. My inner critical voice constantly reminds me of how worthless I am. The fear and shame are a heavy yoke to bear alone. I don't dare confide in anyone.

Suppose Mum dies...

Dad expects loyal silence. I'm not allowed to tell anyone. That would hurt Mum, who's so sensitive. Because my big task is to always protect Mum, I can't say anything that would make her sad. What's more, Dad paints a dreadful picture for me. *'Mum wouldn't like you, if she knew. It would be the end of her.'*

I didn't want Mum to abandon me emotionally even more, and am afraid she might die if I told her. And if Mum dies, perhaps I'll die too... The idea is terribly frightening.

I have a vague memory of trying, at some point during my childhood, to tell someone about the awful stuff that was happening. I don't know who it is, but I remember that I'm not believed. *'It's wicked to invent something like that about other people,'* I'm told. Immediately, the lid goes back on. I feel that I'm the one at fault, and never say anything again.

Several times, Dad threatens to kill me if I tell anyone our dark secret. Silence is the only possible option.

The resignation is like a heavy quilt covering me. The feeling colours my life both at home and at school. I become expert at adapting myself, to the point of forsaking myself. Deep inside me, crying and despair are sealed up in a secret. There's no point in being sad when there's no comfort to be had.

The resigned part of me grows stronger. She feels that life has no purpose. It's pointless to do anything or struggle. All she wants is to die.

Separate worlds

To dampen the anxiety, I develop various compulsive behaviours. I wash my hands over and over again, forever trying to get rid of everything that's happened. The compulsive part of me tries to take control. When I go to bed in the evening, I follow a certain ritual. I have to lie in bed in a particular way, so that I know immediately when my father comes into my room.

That compulsion is a cry for help, but no one understands the signals. Mum lets me be. I can't remember her ever once reacting or acting to protect me or my sister. Does she know what's going on? Does she see, but choose to turn a blind eye? I don't know. I just feel I've been totally abandoned, and I'm certain Mum has to be protected at all costs.

I'm subjected to countless assaults. The situation is unsustainable. I simply can't bear all the suffering. The Little One has to undergo those experiences, that terror, while I keep all the pain out of my everyday conscious state. The Little One experiences the night-time abuse, the hurting body and the pain in her genitals, but the unbearable things are hidden from me.

I protect myself as best I can. Being out of touch with my feelings takes me ever further away from the terrifying part of reality. I live in two parallel worlds. All the pain and horror, shame and guilt are collected in the dark world. In the world of light, the feeling that those terrible things never happened holds sway. They're gone. To cope with being in this world, the other world has to disappear. It's amazing how the mind works. When I was little, that splitting or shutting-down saves me, but in my adult life it becomes a big handicap.

Clever me

In the bright world, I go to school. I enjoy studying and learning new things, but above all I like being praised. For me, achieving is extremely important. Being seen and acknowledged as a high achiever gives me my foothold in this world.

The clever part of me is seen by Mum, Grandpa and my two grandmothers. That feels great, but at the same time not. I become the person they expect me to be. I don't have the strength to be myself.

Externally, my parents keep up fine appearances. No one sees what's going on behind the closed doors of our home. It may sound strange, but we have some happy family times. We do normal things. We're out in the woods, build shelters and pick berries. In the natural environment, everything feels fine.

In the summer, we visit my grandfather's childhood home in the country. It's warm and pleasant, and we bathe in the sea. Gran is very playful. Dad joins in having fun in the water. It feels harmless, thanks to Gran being with us all the time.

In the car on the way home, my sister and I lie on the back seat with a pillow and duvet, and look at the stars in the sky. Dad's driving. Right then, he can't hurt me, and I enjoy the sense of security and peace. But back home in Västerås, life returns to pain and anxiety.

Little white pills

The abuse continues far into my teens. Dad becomes increasingly rough, cold and mean. The rapes often take place in a house far out in the forest. No one hears what's going on. No one can rescue me, and there's nowhere to flee.

It's hard to grasp that Dad, who's so awkward in everyday life, can be so purposeful. But he knows exactly what he's doing. He finds paedophile networks and invites men for group rapes. He spurs the others on, encouraging them to go ever further and move the limits forward. Dad's like a completely different person, alien to me.

I see the grins on the men's faces. Their jeering laughs echo inside my head. While they're partying and drinking I lie there, defeated, waiting. I know it will soon be time for the next round. And I won't get away.

Dad gets pleasure from the violence. I'm terribly scared. When I'm 16 or 17, I resist. I try to break free, and kick against Dad and the other men. But they're too strong, and overpower me. It's degrading, the whole business. To make me docile, Dad drugs me. Those white pills make me feel completely knocked out, without the strength to struggle.

Dad gets increasingly aggressive and violent. He takes a stranglehold on me and is sadistic. He puts rope round my neck and tightens it so that I can hardly breathe. Knives and bottles are used as weapons during the rapes. My attackers are aroused by balancing on the edge, seeing whether I survive or not.

Once, when we're in an apartment with other men, I black out completely. I remember coming to in the bathtub, in the bare bathroom, and realising that they're shouting at me, patting my face, spraying water on me and trying to revive me. They sound scared. Maybe they're afraid I'll die.

Chaos in me

My self-esteem is low. I'm terribly afraid of making mistakes and driven by a strong ambition to perform well. I have to feel approved and clever. Hard work keeps my thoughts busy and helps to fend off memories and feelings.

Now it's the Clever Everyday Teenager who takes me to school, studies and acts normal. She keeps the assaults at bay and doesn't want to know that the other voices in me exist. Completely cut off, she manages what needs to be done.

The Denying One claims that everything is made up, that the abuse has never happened, and the Scornful One accuses Little Joanna — who has experienced the night-time terror — of being weak. Some of the different parts of me know about one another, and often argue. My body has to bear all the pain and fear. It's chaos and pandemonium when they all pull in different directions.

The Angry One truly has reasons to be totally furious. She's the part who's trying to fight her way to freedom. She's strong, but Dad and the other men are stronger. They literally beat her down, crushing her resistance. Afterwards, other parts of me take over completely: a Sad One who's terrified and totally powerless, and a Resigned One who whispers that there's no point in fighting.

Resistance and resignation

The Sad One and the Resigned One are afraid of the Angry One, who frightens the weak ones with her dangerous rage. She causes trouble. When the Angry One resists, the perpetrators become even more violent. The abuse worsens, and it's her fault.

Sometimes the Resigned One — the part of me who's hardly strong enough to exist — seizes control. The only way out, as far as she can see, is to give up completely. For her, death is the only way to escape the suffering. This is unnerving for all the other parts of me. The Resigned One's longing for a horrible end to it all threatens every part's existence.

Then, the Denying One barges in with all her strength and states firmly, *'Surely you realise that what you're talking about never happened. Your own Dad would never be capable of doing that. What a ridiculous, stupid assertion!'*

Frozen fear

Sport becomes my refuge. I play a lot of football. When I'm practising and running, I have an outlet for all my tension. It's a hugely enjoyable feeling, but at the same time about achieving, striving and being the best. I have enormous performance anxiety, knowing I won't be good enough if I don't do my best.

When I'm 20, I met Alf, who in time becomes my great love. Starting a relationship with a guy is a way for me to get away from home and escape. It's a great relief to move out, but the relationship between Alf and me is complicated by my frequent state of acute anxiety.

For me, daring to enter into the feeling of being in love is really difficult. Getting close to someone feels dangerous, and I have a lot of anxiety about sex — a kind of intimacy phobia that cuts me off from myself.

Alf can do whatever he likes with me. As for what I myself want, I have no idea. The obsessive thoughts keep coming and my body gets very tense. Learning just to lie close to him and relax takes a long time. I go on living as best I can.

The Everyday Part of me takes charge of what needs doing. For a few years, I struggle to be a normal adult. The fear and shame are as if frozen deep inside me, but still affect me very strongly. I can't find a solution to the situation.

I defend myself and struggle hard to suppress all the perceptions that trigger the anxiety. But they never disappear. Instead, they live their own life inside me, stealing my strength and impairing my health.

The various parts have widely differing thoughts and feelings about what's happening. They pop out and take over in various situations. I get tired of all the conflicts inside me and don't understand that there are several parts in me.

Internal war

When I'm 24, I leave my boyfriend in Västerås and move to Lund, in the south of Sweden, to study at the university. Living alone is a big change. At home it's so quiet and I can no longer keep the Resigned One in check. I become depressed. My daily life is characterised by anxiety and constant running to fend off all my inner conflicts.

Terrible recollections drub me, in the form of sudden flashbacks. They come at any time and can't be controlled at all. With all my strength, I try to suppress them, but the violence and horrors of the abuse won't leave me in peace. I enjoy studying and try to focus on that. Being busy is a strategy I use to keep my thoughts in order. But in the end, it no longer works. The nasty images push their way to the fore, ever more strongly. I'm overcome by nausea and unable to keep the images away from me.

Sensations that somehow remind me of the abuse make me emotionally relive fragments of dramatic events that have been hidden away. If I see a rape scene in a film, I feel dreadful. Small, simple things set off vile flashbacks. For example, the liquid soap on the toilet looks, feels and smells like semen. That soap makes me want to vomit and I rush out of the bathroom.

A war rages inside me. The smaller parts of me make themselves heard. Other parts protest furiously, shouting at them to stop arguing. That huge struggle goes on constantly inside me. I become very deadlocked in my feelings. Little Joanna and the Denying One argue all the time, while my everyday self tries to function as well as possible. Actually, it's incredible that I manage to keep going in everyday life.

Denial

When I visit Mum and Dad, the part of me that denies the abuse is in control, but as soon as I get back home, I'm totally inundated with flashbacks.

The Denying One is supported by the Scornful One, who makes me feel ashamed. She puts me down completely. *'Is there something special about you or what? God, you feel so sorry for yourself! Doesn't everyone have a hard time sometimes? Pull yourself together!'*

Today, I know the assaults went on from when I was three until my late teens. Dad's betrayal was massive. But Mum, too, was incapable of protecting me throughout my childhood. She didn't see me.

I fight inside and bear the whole burden alone. I don't dare reveal the truth to anyone. I hardly dare spend a single second thinking about the insights that are in me. So, obviously, it's impossible to tell anyone — even Alf. If I tell the truth, no one will be able to like me.

Heavy burden

After my studies, both Alf and I look for jobs in Stockholm, and move there together. My new job at a large company involves demanding tasks. Just as I've become accustomed to doing at school and during my time in Lund, I make big efforts to be good at my work.

I have to present myself as a strong person, and not show how I feel. The running helps me to keep going. I train hard to run a half marathon. With all the tensions in my body, running is my salvation.

But on a ski trip I injure my knee. The pain is severe and, despite surgery and a new ligament, it doesn't get better. Not being able to practise running and relieve the tension is a big loss. My depression worsens and I feel I have no energy.

Now I'm working a tremendous lot, without enjoying my job at all and with no means of running off the frustration. My body aches. Anxiety and fatigue become my constant companions. Eventually, everything catches up with me. Aged 30, I have a burnout.

It feels like I'm carrying my trauma in a rucksack. There, I've collected and stored all my feelings of betrayal and violation. All the pain. Now I no longer have the strength to struggle. The rucksack is far too heavy.

After I've been off sick for a few days, Mum and Dad come to visit me. As soon as I open the front door and let them in, anxiety hits me with catastrophic strength. I collapse on the sofa and literally can't move or say anything. I just lie there. Dad sits down in the armchair next to me and put his hand on me. It's awful. I can barely breathe. Without compassion, Dad pretends he wanted to console me. Mum doesn't understand a thing — just thinks I'm worn down by my job.

Panic anxiety

I stay at home for six months. After the sick leave, I try to return to work, but can't keep it up. I no longer have the strength to keep the parts at a distance. They clamour for attention. Terrible memories keep welling up. They immobilise me and I feel terribly unwell.

Little things, like my boss's hands resembling Dad's, easily spark off the terror. Then the fear becomes so real and dreadful that it's as if I'm suffering abuse over and over again. Rapidly sucked back to the trauma period, I lose touch with reality here and now. Everything around me changes. The room, my physical sensations… I'm small, defenceless and totally alone in the cold, dark room.

The panic attacks make me very tired. The Scornful One shouts, *'You're useless! You don't have the strength to work or exercise. You can't do anything.'* Little Joanna is desperately sad. The Scared One cowers in fright, and the Shame-filled One is intensely, profoundly ashamed to be such a hopeless nutcase.

Somehow, I survive the assaults. I simply have no choice. I don't feel I'm getting any help. I go to counselling sessions, but they focus on my job and work-related stress. No one asks about my childhood, or what's plaguing me.

I'm off sick for ten years. All those years, just dissolving into darkness — it makes my heart heavy with sorrow.

Confused

I seek help from several therapists, but the sessions are muddled and they're at a loss. I seem to be 'too much' for them. My problems are too big and deep. Suddenly, each therapist wants to pull out, and there's a dead halt. Those attempts aren't good experiences for me. I already find it impossible to feel trust after all the betrayals.

Of my own accord, I read books about stress, anxiety and depression. I find a book about mental trauma and immediately recognise myself in its descriptions. Although I know it, I'm still refusing to fully admit to myself that my deep-rooted problems may relate to my childhood.

My fear of what may rise to the surface is strong. I don't want that to happen. During that time, I'm in close touch with my family and have very strong bonds with Mum and Dad.

Visiting my parents at their home makes me confused. Many parts of me know what Dad has subjected me to. Another part of me protests vehemently, shouting that *'Of course it's not true!'*

I'm very preoccupied with conflicting thoughts and feelings and can't moderate all the arguments and friction. A struggle is going on inside me: I'm fighting to survive. None of the parts know it's over — that I'm no longer being abused. It just feels that way. The struggle creates gigantic anxiety.

Safe arms

While I'm off sick, I begin studying to be a counsellor. This leads to more eye-opening discoveries. At the same time, Alf and I are drifting ever further apart.

It's hard to live in the moment. The distance between us keeps growing, and our relationship comes close to ending. Then Alf goes into therapy. I gradually start to feel more loving. I choose him anew, and feel how much in love with him I am.

As my course comes to an end, I overcome the shame and pluck up the courage to tell Alf I've been sexually abused. My body howls with pain, but it's so liberating to finally put it into words. Alf is shocked, but he *believes* me. That's very important. Although I've hidden my dark secrets all these years we've been together, he gives me his full support.

From that day on, Alf's like a steadfast rock. He finds what I've been through terrible, and doesn't really know what to do. But he's *there* for me; he withstands it and takes care of me when I feel bad. I feel very secure. It's wonderful that he can cope with me!

Finally, I come into contact with a therapist specialising in abuse. From her, I get some help in beginning to face my painful family history. Seeing I've been abused, she helps me to accept that I need antidepressant medication.

The therapist notices that I sometimes disappear, and explains that it's a matter of dissociation, but she doesn't tackle my dissociative symptoms. Suddenly, the therapist loses her job and abruptly, in the middle of the process, disappears. Once again, I feel betrayed.

Flame of hope

Now I feel so bad that I seek psychiatric help. The recently qualified cognitive behavioural therapist I meet is unable to help me, but recommends TT. I get in touch. Going into therapy with her makes a huge difference.

All the previous therapists have tried to change me. *'That's enough now, Joanna.'* That was the feeling they've conveyed. They wanted to give me techniques to control my thoughts. *'Don't think like that,'* they would say. But they just scratched the surface, and didn't grasp how divided I was.

TT responds to me in a completely different way, asking novel questions. I want to protect myself, but she stays with what I'm revealing, letting me explore the hard stuff. She affirms my perceptions and helps me understand my own inner reality. At last I'm able to confront the flaming furnace there and fully grasp that I needn't be all alone with my flashbacks and anxiety.

For the first time, I feel confident in a therapist. With her predecessors, my trust has received many blows, and there haven't been any real conclusions. *How can I dare to trust her?* But now I feel understood. TT doesn't think I'm 'odd'; instead, she spots things and takes them seriously. It feels incredibly good to be seen. In our first session, some hope is already awakened in me — hope that there may be a way forward after all. It's life-changing. But it takes time before I venture to trust her all the way.

Vile memories

For me, letting a therapist get really close is a major step. I dare to believe she'll truly stay with me — not abandon or hurt me. We work hard and she shows me how to achieve better equilibrium inside, make sense of what is happening in me and calm down. So the anxiety gradually subsides to some extent.

Eventually, when I've come to trust TT's experience and response to me, I venture into the exploratory process with her. The trust encourages me to open up. Powerful, appalling memories resurface. There's so *much* that has wanted to emerge for so *long*, that needs to get out into the open and be worked through.

At this time, I have no idea there are so many different parts of me. All I know is that there's often total chaos inside, and extreme anxiety set off by the frightening memories that preoccupy me all day long.

The key is to finally be understood, and understand myself, in depth. Today, I know that traumatisation in childhood has resulted in me developing many parts, all with their own distinctive functions, feelings and behaviours. I suppose I've grasped the fact that I dissociate — that I sort of disappear out of myself in the present. After all, I've read about dissociative parts of the personality and am no stranger to such thinking. Still, it's a strange feeling to start getting in touch with my different parts, when they come forward and express various aspects of me. Strange, but still mostly reassuring. I'm becoming more real.

All the parts inside me have different memories. Each one is in its own reality, still living at the time when that particular part emerged. Their ways of dealing with the same situation diverge: they pull in different directions. It's a mess, indeed complete chaos inside me, as long as I don't know anything about the parts. When they argue, disorder rules. After all, we have only one body and they all want to decide what that body is to do and say.

Understanding

All these years, I've been dissociating to avoid feeling chaos and pain. I'm still by no means aware of all the parts inside me. I can't manage them. When my brain dissociates, I retreat to a place that's serene and peaceful. Time is consumed and things get kind of misty for me.

I can be in that state for a long time, but still function reasonably well. It's a mechanism that saved me when I was growing up, but in adult life it creates big problems. My husband notices that I react oddly and sort of recede from the here and now. He says, *'Hello, where did you go now?'* But I don't know...

During the therapeutic process, we explore the various parts of my personality. TT talks to them. They appear and I feel there's something else inside me giving the answers. In some way, it's reassuring that she takes them seriously.

Grasping the truth isn't easy, but gradually I begin to see it. *Who's here now? Who's steering my reactions? How does she think and feel? What does this particular one want?*

As a trained therapist, I have an open view of the mind, but this is hard. I feel lost. The parts can't really be found; still, they come forward with their own thoughts and feelings, wanting different things and using various strategies to deal with difficulties. I alternate between thinking, *What nonsense!* and *That's right!* When TT says my prospects of recovery are good, it gives me hope.

Several of me

The exploration process is intensive. I don't know which parts of my personality make themselves known first, but gradually, one by one, they venture forth. Work on one part leads to contact with another, who then steps forward and becomes increasingly clear.

During the therapy sessions, I have to work on getting in touch with the emotional parts. They perceive that the vile acts are happening in the present, although many years have passed since the physical assaults ended. Everything makes much more sense when I grasp that my reactions in the present are due to what has happened in the past — how this particular part of me is now acting on the basis of her previous experience.

When I perceive a current threat, the Angry One's rage is aroused. The survival alarm goes off. The other parts, unnerved, are cast back into the vileness of the past and feel they're as defenceless as before, when all those dreadful things happened. The sad part of me loses all her strength, whereupon the resigned part — the one who can't take any more and just wants to die — immediately awakens... It's frightening and exhausting for the other parts and me.

TT explains that it isn't at all surprising that I react this way or that. Then the shame subsides and strategies to change the patterns become possible to find. 'Positive thinking' isn't enough. Instead, it's a matter of getting in touch emotionally with the various parts, making them feel they're safe now and the danger is over. They're disconnected with the present when they take over my body and my actions.

Eventually, I'm able to gather all the parts in a circle and make them see and listen to one another. New parts appear as I go along, and are encouraged to come forward. The aim is for everyone to feel welcome to join in and be listened to, talk to the others and be seen.

Sixteen different parts gradually crystallise. Each one receives her own working name. The Angry One, for example, is furious and puts up resistance. The part called the Abandoned One feels totally alone in the world, seen by no one at all. The Scared One, huddled in the dark, hides from every danger. The part we call the Shame-filled One feels disgusted with herself. She's mortified by what the adults have done to her and regards herself as the one at fault. That's far from the whole truth about these dissociative parts, of course.

Perilous rage

Sometimes, the room vibrates with strong feelings. A few parts of my personality are furious with, and mean to, one another. It's an absolute trench war. With TT's help, I'm able to set up protective fences among them. The Angry One's powerful feelings are extremely threatening to the others. The Little, Scared and Abandoned Ones have learnt from Dad's outbursts that anger is highly dangerous. The fences help them feel secure.

The Scornful One resists vigorously. She sees therapy as silly nonsense and thinks I'm suffering a lot of painful experiences for no reason whatsoever. After a tough hour of therapy, the Scornful One may take command, send a text message to TT and announce that I don't want to continue. *'We'll manage better without therapy,'* she states firmly. TT takes such things with equanimity. She understands the drama going on inside me, which is good. I know I need to plunge into those memories and work my way through them, although parts of me are defiant.

The Scornful One can be cruel, not just to therapists but to the other parts as well. She accuses them of being weak and bad, bullies them because they can't cope with anything and calls them totally useless. The Little, Scared and Abandoned Ones believe the Scornful One's nagging, and get upset and frightened. The Little One feels so lousy and useless she goes silent. She's ashamed and feels like a limp, wet rag. She doesn't dare sit and talk to TT when the Scornful One is there, mocking her and saying how pathetic and ridiculous it all is.

Gradually, I come to understand where this pattern comes from. My Dad could be very contemptuous and critical, and in me the Scornful One does exactly the same. Being like Dad is safe. By taking his side, she hopes to avoid being the one who suffers. She follows the one with power. She has learnt that weakness spells danger.

River of sorrow

The therapeutic process becomes a tough inward journey. I keep discovering new 'secrets' kept by a part of me — secrets that, though hidden beneath the surface, rule my life. They've been there all along, demanding attention for ages. Much energy has been devoted to holding them back.

Now that I'm starting to release what's in there, I sense the feelings in my body. It's a necessary requirement for healing. If I begin to disappear, to shut down, TT helps me return to my body.

Over time, my resistance to letting new parts emerge and make themselves heard decreases. Finally, I'm even able to be glad they're coming forward. It would, of course, be a great relief not to have to go through all this: it's incredibly hard, painful work. But now I know it's possible to help them. The realisation that the therapy is genuinely healing me makes it easier to accept it when new parts emerge.

My knowledge of what's in there, in that murky world, grows when the Little One starts appearing more clearly. Simultaneously, a strong part shouts more and more intensively that the vileness never happened. *'It's all just made up,'* nags the voice that denies the Little One's experience and valiantly fights against the truth when it's pulled out into the light.

I'm overwhelmed by resignation. I who want to do so much with my life am now drowning in floods of sorrow and bitterness. The parts' conflicts become obvious. They have such different solutions to everything they can't tolerate.

When the Resigned One takes over my thoughts, there's no point trying to fight. The feeling that things will never get better engulfs me completely. It's hard to handle, because other parts of me are so anxious for a meaningful, wonderful life still to be possible. Life is longing for itself.

For me, it's hard to understand that life can ever be different when it's been so hopeless for so many difficult years. When my sense of resignation becomes too heavy, it's TT who has to sustain the hope.

Dark shame

Apart from all the parts making my mind messy and chaotic, I'm ashamed to have so many voices inside me. I'm burdened by an incredible lot of shame. First and foremost, it's because of what I've been through. I felt so worthless after all the abuse. But I'm also ashamed of having become such a strange person. *All those parts arguing inside me — there must be something wrong with me!*

The more parts you're split into, the more disturbed you are — that's how I feel — and the greater the shame of not being normal.

I'm ashamed of not being able to work properly, too. I want to be good at my job! Like many others who were traumatised as children, I'm driven by a powerful ambition to achieve. First, my fragile self-esteem causes a relentless need for affirmation and approval. Second, the hard work keeps my thoughts busy and helps to keep out memories and feelings. Now that unconscious strategy is no longer effective.

The anxiety makes me infinitely tired. It becomes a vicious circle. In the evening, I find it hard to get to bed, although I long to sleep. One strong part of me is simply too frightened to settle down for the night. The abuse has often taken place in bed at night, after all. Now the terrifying memories are activated when I go and lie down. The violence and powerlessness overwhelm me again and again. The result is even greater exhaustion, even bigger difficulties in coping with my work — and even more shame.

Screaming inside

For a while, terror strikes every morning like a whiplash through my body. Panic seizes me immediately, even before I'm really awake. I'm short of breath, and hyperventilating. My body trembles and shakes. Cold sweat breaks out. I feel chilled and want to get away, but there's nowhere to go. The fear is like a great inner scream, a desperate cry that echoes all through me.

Pain radiates throughout my body. Getting up and moving is unbearable. I weep and almost collapse. Staying upright is difficult. Resignation weighs me down. I can't see how I'll have the strength to go on, to live. I'm paralysed by fear. It feels like I'm dissolving.

I try to calm down, and look around. *Where am I?* I see that I'm in my bedroom — not the old room of my childhood but the one where my adult self is living with Alf. There's no danger here and now. I've been dreaming.

True, I can see where I am, but the fear doesn't let go. Anxiety lurks in my body. At the same time, I'm so tired I don't know how I can get up, let alone get ready, go to work and, once there, concentrate and cope with the pressure. Finally, I take sick leave. All I feel is despair and resignation. Nothing soothes me, although I know there's no danger now, either at home or at work. In fact, everything is fine, but the old stuff still keeps welling up inside me.

Drained and helpless

In the therapy room, I get support in processing the images and strong feelings, all the concrete memories I've kept at bay for so long. I catch my breath and feel how I'm lying there in my bed as a teenager, and how Dad bends down over me, spreads my legs and forces himself on me, shoving his way into my vagina, inflicting unbearable pain.

I sense how the revulsion and terror fills me. My whole body shakes violently. I cry, snort and breathe heavily, wanting to get away. Panic-stricken, I begin to kick and hit out. My legs want to kick, my arms to break free, and I try to get him off my body. When it's happening, in reality and my flashbacks, I can't protect myself. He's too heavy and strong. There's no getting away. But now, when I relive it in the therapy room, I'm able to defend myself. And my body wants it — oh, how much it wants to move!

Reliving the assaults is physically painful. Intense pain radiates into my stomach and my whole back. I double up and pull my legs to my chest, wailing loudly. I feel cramp in my genitals, and almost stop breathing. TT sees to it that I take a break, keep breathing and rest frequently.

I want to get out of there, but stay. I see his face and body so close — too close. I hear him groan, feel him thrust. He's enjoying it — my own father, with me. It's so repulsive I just want to vomit.

When he's done, it's as if nothing has happened. *'Now you've got to hurry,'* my father says. He's going to give me a lift to school. But I remain lying there. Used. Disgusted. Resigned. Deathly tired. How can I find the strength to get up? Get dressed, have breakfast, sit in the car next to him, be at school and concentrate? How will I be able to pull myself together? Listen and function during lessons? All I want is to die and escape from it all. There's nothing to look forward to.

There in the therapy room, I relive it all — all the feelings and bodily sensations I've borne inside for so long. My body is sore. I feel drained and helpless. Where there should be strength, there's nothing left but fear and resignation. But it's worked; the sense of relief always follows a stint of hard work. Serenity comes, and I can leave the therapy feeling several kilos lighter.

Finding my strength

After the outburst in the therapy room, it's crystal-clear that those are precisely the feelings that have overwhelmed me every morning for the past few months — and long before that. There I lie now, weak and exhausted, and empty and light inside. The kind of deep work I've done today in the therapy room vibrates throughout my body. Now comes the wonderful sense of relief. Some weight inside me — a heavy burden I've carried my whole life — has gone. I'm filled with feelings of joy, almost happiness. And now there's no pain whatsoever in my body — just tranquillity and peace.

After that, the mornings are nowhere near so fraught. The hard times don't stop altogether, but there's a great difference. My intense anxiety, terror and panic on waking are almost completely gone. I feel calmer, more present here and now. Things feel nowhere near as tough and unpleasant, and my despondency and resignation are gone. Facing the day ahead feels okay — even good sometimes. Joyful.

The Sad Teenager is here and now more, and much less restless than before. She feels calmer and less scared. Although she occasionally goes back to the trauma period, she's in the present much more. She knows and senses that it's peaceful and safe now, that times have changed and life is no longer a constant ordeal, as it was when she was growing up. She's successively grasping the fact that she's living in a time and place where there's no abuse, no longer a need to fight and endure, and no more incessant pain. Now, here, she's safe and enjoying good things: Alf, the cats and a secure home with warmth, joy and consideration. It's bewildering to her, but she's slowly beginning to see the world we're living in now. Her flashbacks are becoming less frequent and, above all, she's able to start communicating with the other two teenagers.

She has borne the pain for so many years. Now she has related — and all the parts know — what happened. She has performed an incredibly hard task. All the others are helping and looking after her now. The Sad Teenager is close to me now. I embrace her.

Before, I may have known that things weren't too bad here at home or at work. But she didn't know that: she was still in the past, kept there by the terror, feeling acutely lonely and despondent. Now, she can also be in the present, looking around, taking it in and feeling. The more she's here, the more all the parts are here, the more serene I become inside and the more

I can relax. An enormous weight inside me is being lifted from every cell in my body. I feel liberated.

From darkness to light

Strong feelings still get going when, for example, there's a stimulus from outside. During my flashbacks, these feelings take over. They appear with great speed, flooding me with fear and making me want to escape.

When I see on the TV news that a woman has suffered a group rape on a ferry to Finland, I'm swept away in a cold darkness. The whole world around me turns black. My body tenses up, I feel surrounded by danger and I shake with fear.

Slowly I begin to acquire tools that help me deal with the anxiety attacks. In the therapy, we work on memories from when I myself was gang-banged. The powerlessness, the pain, the scornful laughter, the petrifying fear... all the vile abuse my body and soul have been through, which I've carried deep inside me... are now finally emerging.

Afterwards, I'm exhausted and somewhat out of it, but then a powerful sense of relief washes over me. I'm *here* again — back in the moment. I feel my body relaxing. A warm light enfolds me. It's superb that trauma processing makes such a huge difference. Joy grows inside me.

New tools

I have no idea of when or how I've developed the various parts of my personality. For a long time, having several parts of me feels very troublesome and disorderly. *Who feels what? Who's saying this? Who's that, expressing this feeling? Who wants this, in particular?*

Sometimes, when all the parts are active, chaos rules inside me. Contradictory thoughts and feelings clash. Opinions and beliefs about what has actually happened and how I should live my life are sharply divided. Still, in time the various parts are becoming clearer — to one another, too. The sense of inner chaos is slowly subsiding. Step by step, I seem to be moving towards recovery, and these changes are revolutionary for me. Little by little, I'm beginning to believe in a different life from the one I've had so far.

Now I dare to see the wounded parts of myself. Everything is becoming more manageable as my awareness of who's saying what grows and I increasingly understand where the various feelings belong.

I'm building bridges

I'm gradually learning to take in the various voices without being completely sucked into their emotional ebbs and flows. When the parts who have lived in the dark world feel they are listened to, they no longer need to be so scared and aggressive. My work and daily life are going ever more smoothly; the medication doses I have to take are constantly decreasing; and my physical pain — though still partially there — is lessening too. When I was off sick before, I wasn't able to do any running at all for nine long years. Now I'm starting to manage it again. It's a wonderful feeling.

The emotional parts have a range of different reactions and feelings. Often, one of them has dominated my body, actions and speech with her will. Now I know they exist and are capable of seizing control of me. Before, they haven't known about one another. They have all been running their own races, and felt very lonely. Through therapy, we're getting the parts to cooperate and turn inwards to one another instead of isolating themselves in their solitary struggles. This recognition is vital. Now I'm beginning to understand that there's no need for them to work against one another.

The emotional parts are still reacting as they've been in the habit of doing for many years, but not pulling as hard in different directions. This cooperation represents major progress. In the group, they no longer feel so lonely. When they're seen and listened to, I sense them becoming more secure and starting to relax. I feel more composed.

The Silent One, who has been mute and shy, becomes more secure when she notices she is not the only part who is scared and sad. Now she no longer needs to use her silent strategy: instead, she's beginning to express herself. Meanwhile, the Abandoned One no longer needs to bear the burden of all that fear of rejection alone. Formerly like islands in an endless sea, they're beginning to connect through mutual support and consolation. They know about, feel fellowship with and help one another. Compassion is emerging. Now I'm increasingly calm.

Into the warmth

The three teenagers, who have borne such different issues, are approaching one another. The Sad Teenager, who is so depressed and still lives in the terrible old days, is discovering she is no longer alone. Before, she knew nothing of the others; now, slowly, she's daring to believe there are others who can support her. In the therapy, she's helped to leave the menacing life in the old family house behind her, walk away and step into our safe home, where Alf and I live. Here in the warmth, she's finally able to be an ordinary teenager and start mourning what she's missed out on. Sometimes, the Sad Teenager forgets that she exists here and now, but then the Angry Teenager helps, showing her how safe it is here. This gives the Sad Teenager new hope and strength to live.

It may sound strange to someone who has never experienced anything of the kind, but there may be room for many parts in a person, and there is no pretending this is not so. Now that mine have started being together, getting to know one another and their respective situations, mutual help works. Before, the Sad One was unaware of her two peers. The Angry One knew about the Sad One but thoroughly detested her and her weakness, and tried to chase her away. The Everyday Teenager wanted nothing to do with either of the other two and was afraid of the Angry One.

Pain of denial

A key feature of the treatment is the training I've been able to do at home. TT makes short recordings that I can listen to daily. This practice, or training, creates continuity and enables me to make progress on my own. Not everything hinges on my sessions with TT. The recordings help me soothe myself, bring my parts more into the here and now and help us avoid judging one another and ourselves. She calls it 'compassion training'. Her voice guides me in the task of assembling all my parts and working further on them on my own. This is a great boon in the summer when she's on holiday, and makes the break less arduous.

After two years' therapy, life starts to go better. The Resigned One has less influence than before. As I work on what activates her, I find ways to do things differently.

The part of me that finds it hardest to embrace the therapy is the Scornful One. Getting her on side, working for our progress, is exceptionally complicated and difficult. She's been so powerful and harsh, like a mini-Dad in me. Now that she sees him as he is and knows what the other parts have gone through, she feels tender towards them. Inducing the Scornful One to change her attitude is a tough job, but now she hardly ever pours scorn any more. On the contrary, she's usually friendly and appreciative towards the others.

The part who has denied that the abuse happened has also been a tough nut to crack. Finally, she can even admit that Dad really did force me to commit incest. Now, that part is small and very tired. She can join us in the circle, but can't boss the others around or put them down. I see that denial is the message from my parents that I've taken over as my own. Dad and Mum resolutely claim that the abuse never happened. That I've made it all up.

Family ties

Sometimes I feel angry about the hell I was forced to live in as a child, but also about the heavy impact it's had on my whole life. The feeling of being different, never being safe, not having a family to hang out with — it inflicts real damage on a person, in many ways.

Nowadays, I'm no longer in touch with my parents, siblings, grandmother, nephews and nieces. It saddens me, and still feels a bit unreal, that my family have chosen to turn their backs on me. But the truth has set me free. For me, daring to remain standing — not give way, or let myself down — is something great.

Today, I'm still unsure how my sister was affected during our childhood. I always tried to protect her and take the knocks as far as I could, so that she would escape.

I miss my siblings. My sister has closed the door on me. I used to be in close touch with her son; now I've disappeared from his life. That hurts. What is he to think? And my brother has had children I've never met. Standing up for myself has major consequences. I can't be there for Gran now that she's undergoing arduous cancer treatment.

Inside me, there's a yearning for my mother to be here, believe in me and give me hugs. At times like Christmas, New Year's Eve and birthdays, the wish is especially acute. I've longed for my family, but to get well I've needed to get out of their grip and break the destructive patterns. It's worth it to avoid living in the old lies.

Love and lust

Now I'm 44 and have succeeded in returning to my job. I'm working half-time and I enjoy having the energy to cope with it. True, I'm very tired after work, but I can still live a fairly ordinary life. I can do the housework, wash up and go shopping without being so stressed out and exhausted that I start dissociating. It's been a great relief to be able to manage simple everyday tasks.

For six years, I've been married to Alf, my childhood sweetheart. Only when we were engaged to be married did I dare to feel really in love.

Before, I could feel love but still found it difficult to achieve closeness, and allow myself to really *feel* for him. Physical intimacy aroused much sorrow in me and I kind of ended up somewhere else. For several years, we couldn't make love. It's incredible that my husband has coped with it, and stayed with me.

In the past year, there's been a breakthrough. I feel secure with Alf and myself. I'm capable of being here and now, relaxing and enjoying life more. We're intimate and I enjoy it — my desire and my feelings, everything. At last, I'm allowing myself to be in love!

Longing for children

I yearn intensely for all I'd missed. Above all, I long to feel more strength and energy — to be able to live an ordinary life and have a sense of well-being — and to have children. Should we dare to try, or is it already too late, perhaps?

One day, on discovering I'm pregnant, I'm overwhelmed with joy. To protect the child, I promptly stop taking almost all the medication. In particular, the effects of going without two strong drugs I've been taking for over a decade are clearly noticeable. Suddenly, my body feels even more of what I've found unbearable before. The aching affects me a lot. With crawling sensations in my body, it's hard to sit or lie still. But I can handle it. I think about the tiny being who is to be our child.

Sadly, the pregnancy ends in a miscarriage. That hard blow makes me lose my footing. Suddenly, I'm thrown into icy darkness. I find myself feeling cold, shaking and crying. Irrational anxiety is triggered with full force, and holds me in a vice-like grip. My body, which has already experienced so much pain and powerlessness, is petrified of all the new things that are happening. Again, I have to go on full-time sick leave.

The child parts of me don't understand what's happening at all. They're completely trapped in the fear of dying, of being annihilated. In the therapy room, a lot of work is needed to explain to the little ones what has happened.

A relief to mourn

Before the miscarriage hit us, all my parts were integrated most of the time. When TT asked me to estimate how much of my waking time I felt I was a whole person, my answer was about 70 per cent. That was a great leap forward. Now, after the miscarriage, the shock has revived the various parts, each of whom reacts in her own way and pulls in her own direction. That's a big setback. The Resigned One takes up a lot of space and sucks the strength out of me.

Recovering my balance takes time. However, the work slowly progresses. Every part of me is bravely striding forward. The therapy process really makes a difference and the certainty gives me the strength to keep working.

It's a relief when the tears come, and liberating when the grief is expressed. Now, all the parts can sit down together and feel they're not alone, and are helping one another. I relax, which is a great feeling. And I can cope without returning to the old medication. The pregnancy and miscarriage mean that new recovery work can start, and it also deepens the previous results. My progress is much faster than in the work I've done before. My understanding of the parts — their origins and reactions — becomes even more obvious to me. We come much closer to one another.

Here and now

A crucial aspect of the therapeutic work has been fully realising that the traumatic experiences belong to the past. That the abuse isn't happening over and over again. That they can no longer hurt me.

I've learnt to disconnect the past and present. Before, it was difficult or impossible to relax and enjoy, to just be in the moment. The fear from the past, which still dominated me, could flare up at any moment and sabotage my perception of the present. I *knew* I was fine, but it didn't *feel* that way at all. Various parts of me were still terrified, simply because of the many vile things they had experienced, and remained in the old, terrifying reality. In the past, it was like that all the time. It's impossible to describe how awful it was. Now there's something else too. The more I learn mindfulness and acceptance, the more my parts can stay in the present. They've all created a different basic attitude to one another: a non-judgemental one. It's like a whole new view of myself — of everything and everyone else too, in fact.

I've developed the ability to soothe myself. Now I recognise what's happening and know what I can do to manage my feelings.

Living life

During the therapeutic work done jointly with TT, I've come into contact with the force that wants to live and create. I've started painting again and I've had an exhibition. It's wonderful to be creative, be able to make art and discover that I can feel peaceful at the same time.

Feelings of contentment now arise spontaneously and bring relaxation, which is a whole new experience for me — someone as tense as a bowstring in the past.

Because of my intense anxiety, I used to need eight different medicines, which affected me a lot. Now, I'm almost medication-free and can manage completely without sleeping pills.

Mothering myself

For a long time, I was unconsciously terrified that everything would fall apart if I allowed myself to have fun and wasn't on my guard. So I was extremely tense. After being unable to run for 16 years, I'm now really enjoying the training. I'm building up my stamina and getting stronger, have more energy and am happier.

I'm driven by the hope of being fully understood, with all my parts visible. They all now know what's happened. It can still be messy and fragmented at times, but now it's possible to gather them all. They can be close to one another. The terrible things that happened then, long ago, don't take over. Mutual trust is growing.

The Resigned One has found her joy and is discovering that life can be wonderful without everything suddenly being ruined. The Clever One, who has long been driven by the compulsion to achieve, feels freer and more creative. She's no longer afraid of making mistakes or being wrong.

Step by step, I'm approaching an everyday life in which all the parts have merged into one, where there's space for all their experiences and they're integrated. Sometimes it's a bit messy. It gives me loads of work and I can get so tired of the parts and their fuss, but when I find a way that works, I realise I'm developing my leadership. There was never a secure adult in their lives. Now, I'm like a parent to my inner children. A good parent!

Now, I experience long periods when there are no separate parts at all. Then comes the payoff: I'm really alive, like other people — serenely whole, with no fragmentation. During a concert, I may suddenly think, *Oh, where IS everyone? What does everyone think?* Then I relax and trust we're one.

At work, I'm now usually fully integrated. With all the parts united here and now, I know better what I need and feel where my boundaries are. That makes me secure. I dare to say no to the boss. *'That's enough now,'* I say calmly. Then he backs down. Everything feels more enjoyable; I have the energy to tackle things and get pleasure from successfully completing slightly more complicated tasks. Nothing needs to be perfect: good enough is okay. For me, that's something new.

Truth heals

Although the memories remain in me, they don't affect me as they used to do. The difference is that I've lived through the experiences. They're like other memories — not charged with emotion — and so don't steal my energy.

My whole life's different now. I can have an adult approach. Of course, it's deeply unfair that I was subjected to incest and denial; that's a double betrayal. But at least *I* take myself seriously. I *have* in fact experienced all that vile stuff. It's really *too* awful for a single child to be subjected to that. But that's the way it is.

When I dare to talk about my childhood, I get strong reactions. Some people find it hard to take in the fact that abuse happens. They don't want to see all the pain and ill health that the exploitation leads to. There are so many fears. Many people probably still think that you shouldn't reveal anything about family secrets. Strangely enough, there's more concern for the perpetrator than the victim. But why should I, who have been subjected to violence and total powerlessness, protect adults who have done wrong?

Actually, I don't want to hang out with my Dad. I'm ashamed for his sake, because he did what he did and is as he is. Besides, I want to protect Mum, not show her in a bad light. But they live far away and we have no contact. Taking up space and telling my story has a healing effect on me. My parents can live as they please. I'm not able or willing to share their world of lies.

The sweetness of freedom

Never again will I accuse myself or put myself down for what I was subjected to. And I want never again to be ashamed because it made me ill.

For me, it was a great relief that I had a dissociative disorder, both for getting the right treatment and for my self-esteem. It's truly reassuring to know why I've been functioning in that strange way. I was so resigned and could never believe that change was possible. Hearing *'Your difficulties are fully possible to work on and have a very good prognosis'* felt wonderful. And it was true, because today I no longer have that diagnosis.

Now I understand why the rapes were shut off from my everyday self. It may sound odd, but how else could I have got by in daily life, gone to school and simultaneously coped with what was happening at night and other times? That reality was so dangerous, so full of pain and terror, shame and guilt, that shutting down became my only way out.

It's incredible how cleverly the human psyche works. When I was little, the division into several parts was my salvation. But then it started ruining my adult life, although the abuse had stopped and I was actually able have a good life.

As my recovery process has continued, the whole of me has realised that all the hard times are over. We've put a proper distance between ourselves and all that old stuff. We can look through the same eyes, see and experience the same things and breathe at the same time. We smile at the same things. We know we're safe.

Before, not all the emotional parts knew that. They were cut off from one another on their separate islands. Some time ago, I was still sometimes able to discern the islands, but now I walk around as a single, whole person on a solid continent.

Little by little, in this new security, we've merged into me, and I'm extremely grateful that I finally received the right help. That I was able to be off sick when I needed to be, and didn't have to work to survive, and that public services provided psychotherapy for me. Now I'm working, taking my place in society and am largely medication-free. Soon, I'll give birth to my baby. Just think — that this is possible! I feel the movements and kicks, and have seen an ultrasound image of how the foetal heart is beating and how it's practising breathing. That moves me so much. Humbly, I'm filling up with the best things in life. That tiny being — the sweetest little human in the world, of course! — is wonderful to see. There are really no words to describe what being free from my past is like. I'm alive and well, like an ordinary person.

I feel that I'm creating my new world here, now, today. I'm living a normal life. Nothing haunts me, restricting my life, and there's no deep fissure in my soul. There's space for every feeling inside me. I'm whole: a whole person. Loved and free.

I'll never forget the vileness, but it can no longer hurt me. I know who I am, and I deserve to live a blissful life here on Earth. I've struggled hard to achieve this sense of well-being. With help, I succeeded and now I can enjoy all the beauty that exists in this world.

CHAPTER 13

The whole person needs help

Trauma wounds can genuinely destroy survivors' whole existence. To achieve success in the therapy room we need, as noted in previous chapters, to strive for a meeting of equals between patient and therapist. Together they form a team that, with joint forces, work to achieve the common goal: for the patient to attain ever greater self-awareness and a sound, happy life.

Trauma-related dissociation is far from easy to understand. It locks in parts of the mind, makes life chaotic and generates immense suffering. How can professional practitioners proceed when faced with hard-to-treat, complex conditions like dissociative disorders? In this chapter, we explore the many challenges of therapeutic work.

Dissociation: simultaneously knowing and not knowing

Having experiences that are not fully integrated is something that, of course, happens to us all. But if this is a recurring phenomenon during childhood, a serious deficiency arises. *'Dissociation involves a kind of parallel owning and disowning of experience: While one part of you owns an experience, another part does not'* (Boon et al., 2011).

For the victim, unsuccessful integration gives a continuous perception that *not all my experience is my own; some of it belongs to someone else*. The sense of self is fragmented and incoherent, rather than enduring.

Dissociative syndrome or disorder is structural in nature — that is, not a temporary condition or isolated incident. Subsystems that are insufficiently integrated have arisen. As noted in previous chapters, two main groups of dissociative parts of the personality (aspects of the person) are usually created. These are the everyday (apparently normal personality, ANP) parts and the survival (emotional personality, EP) parts.

As you may remember, EP parts are usually of a victim or controlling nature. Those in a strong position of control work hard to be in charge, and devote much energy to this behaviour. Not infrequently, there is conflict and the controlling figure takes command by fighting for its existence. The primary characteristic of the parts of a victim nature is that they are highly vulnerable. They try to survive by submission and avoidance.

Everyone must join in

In successful treatment, all the parts *must* join in the work. They all need to feel that the therapist sees, recognises and respects them. Understanding this inner structure of people with complex traumatisation is something of a fundamental theme to learn about in psychotherapeutic work with the severely traumatised. The therapist's question is: *What is this structure like in the person now in front of me?*

Since every part is filled with its own memories and feelings, they may have widely differing treatment needs. Their degrees of motivation for wanting to participate in the therapy may also vary, and can change during the process. Initially, some may not want to attend at all. When one part feels relief about the diagnosis, another may react with anger or denial. If a part's survival strategy has long been based on keeping all the awful events secret, being 'found out' is terrifying.

Strong fear and a power struggle among the parts are real challenges. If the therapist falls into the trap of forming an alliance with survival parts of a victim nature, the healing process comes to a halt. The victim side is vulnerable and easy for us, the caregivers, to like. Controlling parts are easily seen as merely putting up resistance — behaviour that will mature and disappear. These parts may therefore not even have been allowed to take part in the treatment, and been simply rejected as just representing negative behaviour that the patient must learn to refrain from. This pattern in the treatment work must be stopped. It is simply essential to include parts of a controlling nature in the therapeutic work as well.

Warning

Controlling parts of the personality, as much as others, have their own trauma memories that need working through. Behind a part's need for control hides its vulnerability, in need of healing. In this part, rage and other strong forces are central. If controlling parts are left out of treatment, destructive behaviours easily increase instead of gradually disappearing. At worst, this can have disastrous consequences. Splitting among the various parts often then becomes even more profound.

This can lead to a never-ending struggle with, for example, suicide attempts or suicide threats, long periods of self-harm or outbursts of sudden externally directed rage. At the same time, parts may develop even greater weakness, with an emphasis on vulnerability. The outcome can be a severe deadlock in the patient, which rules out recovery.

With the best of intentions, we can all treat patients without understanding what they are communicating to us. Powerful therapeutic methods that otherwise work well can become our ways of filling the treatment sessions, either without any great success or, at worst, to the detriment of the severely traumatised patient.

Arduous process

Post-traumatic stress disorder (PTSD) means that the symptoms have not healed after one or more traumas. Focused work is required to remedy the wounds that are left behind. Sometimes, patients are unwilling to do that work. They are content to have survived and accept the option of going on living with certain consequences and symptoms. If so, they need to be respected for this decision.

However, traumatised people often want help or perceive that they need it to make progress. They no longer have the strength; their everyday lives are affected too much, and are full of stress, insomnia, anxiety, depression of the PTSD type, dissociation and more. Then, they must be able to get help with the consequences of the traumatisation in particular.

Regardless of the degree of traumatisation, the healing requires work, unless the problem itself abated after the difficult event(s). Others sometimes express a romanticised wish that the solution must be to meet a new partner. Finding love again, they think, would solve the problem and bring back happiness. We tend to think, wishfully, that hard work should not be necessary. We may hope that a new job, a new home, new love or some other external change is the answer.

Finding love or making other changes may be entirely right and wonderful. It may make things easier for us but, as such, does not end the post-traumatic state. Nevertheless, we humans may subsequently explain, to ourselves or in response to pressure from others, that our recovery from PTSD is due to precisely these visible external changes in our lives. But if one has undergone an arduous process and worked hard to get through personal trauma, one should acknowledge the good efforts one has made, rather than ascribing the causes of the improvement to external circumstances, and be proud of that good, hard work.

Every symptom needs treating

As we all know, the diagnosis itself solves no problems. The right treatment must also be offered, and the purpose of the diagnosis should be to ensure adequate treatment. In the care services, we cannot just diagnose traumatisation and then forget, or decide to skip, the requisite work.

Traumatisation, irrespective of its degree of severity, cannot just be identified in a patient and then not treated, or treated only with psychotropic drugs and other medication. Nor is it enough to treat only one or two of the post-traumatic symptoms, such as depression or insomnia, and exclude the others and their repercussions. Treating just a few symptoms can improve the patient's condition only very marginally, both in extent and over time. This does not mean that medication may be unnecessary, or that depressive disorders or sleep problems should be ignored. But along with the other consequences of traumatisation, the problems need to be treated.

Today, unfortunately, the victims themselves are often obliged to push for, pursue and demand treatment for their traumatisation. All too often, their words fall on deaf ears. Many survivors end up in unreasonable vicious circles in the healthcare system. They are often treated for depression, anxiety or bipolarity, while other post-traumatic tribulations and symptoms are not even noticed. Correct, adequate help is not forthcoming, and the traumatisation is often not identified at all.

Key crossroads for therapists

Many of us professionals who work with traumatised people see clearly that we need to acquire far more knowledge and experience of the various conditions involved, especially those involving a high degree of dissociation. We never learn all there is to know. The less we know, the more we risk harming the traumatised.

Thus, before we begin psychotherapeutic treatment, the degree of dissociation needs to be identified and diagnosed as far as possible. The less dissociation there is, the sooner tackling the trauma itself is advisable. The higher the degree of dissociative disorder, the more the victim needs help to gain stability. The initial emphasis of the treatment then needs to be on stabilisation. This is sometimes confused with supportive counselling, which is different.

The skills training required in stabilisation work must be adapted to the person's degree of traumatisation. A well-trained therapist can tailor the stabilisation phase to the individual. Some parts of the treatment can be provided in groups. At the end of this book there are facts about group manuals and recommendations on their use. There are manuals for treating both patients with complex PTSD and those with dissociative disorders.

Compassion

Learning to understand trauma-related dissociation is tricky. Trauma therapists' process of taking in what the victim communicates and connecting it with their theoretical knowledge is a complicated one. The task of mindfully perceiving how all the system's different participants express their respective wants is challenging, but also immensely rewarding. This does not mean that we invariably succeed.

Why is it so difficult? As we know, every individual's narrative style, experience and inner dynamics are distinctive. Everyone has a unique network of neural connections in the brain and a vast number of signals passing to and fro between body and brain that are not exactly the same as in any other living being.

But we need to see patterns, listen at many levels and help create scope for inner balance, and successively subdue the devastating, ever-active internal critic. Gradually, we create access to compassion within the survivor.

In people with many dissociative personality parts, this may be a huge challenge. In separate self-constructions that vary within and among the parts, they have created the various worlds they inhabit. Their perceptions of their own egos may fluctuate greatly, resulting in highly diverse behaviours on different occasions. Sometimes information seeps through among them, sometimes not. Some parts may cooperate closely, but also shun one another. An emotional part may fill the others with terror.

Sometimes, they are unaware of one another's existence. That is where we begin the work... and we need to create a team.

Building bridges

As noted above, we are all biopsychosocial beings. We constantly react biologically, psychologically and socially in a complex interplay. This means that we cannot exist solely as one or the other side of ourselves: no side would exist without the others. Structural dissociation brings this to a head. All the parts are right, but limited. They need one another, but probably have no understanding of this at all. Like all the rest of us, they have a compelling need to have kind people around them. But since the people in their vicinity have been dangerous, the survivors have not been able to exist in the kind of peaceful interplay that is required for personality integration and healthy relationships with others.

We therapists need to help our patients understand themselves and work on their own subsystems. We also need to support their development into a team and creation of a world based on compassion and respect among the parts of the personality. With greater compassion, sense of security and respect in the inner system, the world can look a little less threatening in there. The fear or terror that lies in the air among the parts calms down a little. At best, chances of changing perspective gradually increase. As a result, we can then work on the traumatising experiences and, in the long run, integrate all our subsystems.

Destructive acts

We need to help the parts begin to reflect. When we understand their functioning in the system, we can work to calm down their constant 'substitute actions'. These form behaviour patterns that the parts have had to acquire earlier in life to divert pain and suffering — unpleasant experiences they have had no control over.

Such substitute actions can become highly problematic for people when, later in life, they are no longer in danger — when, for example, strong feelings become overwhelming, or when a part has been truly activated and ends up with the perception of having returned to the old, past situations. The old way of trying to cope with it may then be the way in which the part acts again. The actions may include a wide range, from physical self-harm to not eating and otherwise exposing oneself to danger.

They are not infrequently resorted to repeatedly, not because the person wants to return to the past but because there is a deep-seated hope that the outcome will be different this time.

The therapeutic work cannot be completed without such actions cropping up during the process. However, every time they are activated, progress can usually be made, and recurrence becomes less likely. Finally, the behaviour is gone. It is important to understand that every substitute action should, for a person who needs it, be not just eliminated but replaced by a sounder coping strategy.

Responding to the victim role

Thus, we cannot treat the parts separately. Tackling their interrelationships — that is, the whole system — is necessary. We must work to promote internal communication. As one patient put it, *'It feels like I have a whole pre-school group inside me. I have to teach them all to sit down in the circle and listen to one another.'*

First, we need to focus on the cognitive level and then proceed to the emotional level. When we work on thoughts, we are working to promote understanding and insight and combat self-destructive accusations. In various ways, we provide practice in keeping a certain distance or space to train the patient's ability to think and act less impulsively, rather than being caught in the old pitfalls and patterns. We help the patient to practise soothing, stabilising behaviours and thoughts. This can be done by head or eye movements, breathing or other physical exercises. What can help them in a specific situation? Usually, becoming able to unwind at moments of duress means that freedom grows and joy arises. This joy frequently surprises the patient, and very often pride shines through. *'I can do it!'* Feelings of powerlessness are diminished, imparting a sense of freedom.

When we then proceed to work at the emotional level, there is a more stable foundation to stand on — something patients have often never had before. One dissociative part perceives danger, has a sense of panic and frightens itself with thoughts of horrors to come. The tornado of feelings picks up speed and strength. Terror spreads to other parts and the chaos prevails. All the parts have their own solutions for how to save themselves and an extremely hard struggle about what to do ensues.

The ability to remember what must be done to calm oneself is needed when, further on in the therapy, painful feelings and memories need to be worked through. In the treatment room, the therapist can help, give reminders and find ways. To cope in the painful process of reliving memories stored in the body, patients need to use myriads of tricks and method. They also need to do a great deal of work on their own between sessions.

Step by step

As noted several times above, hard work is required for a survivor to attain a healthy life. But taking one step at a time gives a vital sense of improvement during the process. When the therapy starts, it is often a great challenge for the patient to remember what happened during the treatment session. Listening to a recording of the session can then be very helpful. Other examples are various exercises to stay stable. Making everyday life increasingly workable, with all that needs to be done and arranged, also requires great deliberate effort. Further work is also needed to practise mindfulness and self-compassion.

Training in facing up to other parts and practice in cooperation come a bit further on in the treatment. Working to improve and change close relationships with others usually calls for substantial efforts, as does finding employment if this is relevant but has not been achieved previously.

Triggers and traumatic memories should not be what governs either the patient's everyday life or the therapeutic quest for recovery. We therapists need to make an effort not to accompany the affected on unconscious emotional rollercoasters that plunge them into severe anxiety attacks. Our responsibility is to ensure that work in the therapy room remains balanced, and that frequent chaotic emotional releases do not take place. Instead, feelings should be processed at a pace and intensity level that are manageable for the traumatised person.

Phases of trauma therapy

Patients with trauma-related dissociation can be successfully treated with the theory of phase-oriented trauma-focused psychotherapy as a well thought-out foundation. Psychotherapists who work with this patient group on this basis develop this excellent platform and method in slightly different ways, integrating the procedure and making it their own. It is multifaceted and subtle work, adapted to the individual, and must be created in teamwork by the patient and therapist in their sessions.

The first phase emphasises that victims need help to achieve stabilisation and regain some serenity where necessary; overcome their 'attachment and separation phobia'; and master their frequently strong avoidance of all mental and bodily activities, such as feelings, thoughts, desires and fantasies. In particular, patients need to defeat the phobia of being in their own body and facing all their dissociative parts.

How can we understand the functions of these parts in the system? Do any of them serve as an internal safety valve? Which ones are involved when what happens? What are their mutual relationships like? What needs exist to have the parts separated from one another? This is a solid, comprehensive task for the patient and psychotherapist jointly. All further work rests on the outcome of this phase's achievements.

The parts' tug-of-war

In the second phase, exploration of attachment and separation difficulties needs to be continued and intensified. The trauma therapist needs to establish contact with the emotional parts and be in touch with the traumatic level at which they are located. Here, too, the traumatic ties between the perpetrator and the patient's various parts are an important topic.

Now it is even more important for the therapist to develop personal relationships with the various parts, while fostering broader cooperation among them. The starting point is their desire to deal with situations in completely different ways. This generates constant conflicts, anxiety and tugs-of-war about who should be in charge. Sometimes, work in the therapy room resembles efforts made to reduce conflicts among school classmates or siblings, or at a workplace. It requires courage, honesty and understanding both of one's own and of others' reactions, feelings and actions.

We humans often have reasons for acting as we do that are beyond our own comprehension, and our mode of functioning is fundamentally much the same. Here, we therapists may need to work hard to avoid sweeping problems under the carpet and failing to address important issues with the patient, since this may mean that we empower one part or become too dominant and controlling ourselves. The process must take its course, just like when we build truly secure group relationships among people. The parts need to agree not to hurt one another, nor to harm the body they all share.

In this phase, it is also important to work on the patient's avoidance (often described as 'phobic') of the traumatic memories. The memories that constantly blight daily life can be worked on in orderly ways, cognitively and emotionally, in this phase. The parts often have divergent memories, and seldom want to hear about one another's. All the parts find bearing their own enough, although they do not see them as memories at all but as current events, constantly going on. In this phase, the work shifts from stabilisation to collaboration among parts — that is, exposure to traumatic memories. This means revisiting the memory while having a secure foothold in the present. The goal for all the parts is to identify themselves as members of a collective community.

Balancing act

There is no need for patients to be exposed to memories that are not disturbing to them, but these memories may be helpful in other ways. They provide information about the patient's life at the time when the traumatising events were taking place. Patients always show the way by conveying information through their behaviour — a narrative that expresses itself in many different ways. The memories convey what is unfinished and cannot be left behind by the patient without work. Sometimes, they are just bodily memories that do not reach the conscious mind, but which need to receive their due, adequate space and attention.

Assessment of how these memories should be exposed requires responsiveness and communication with the victim's entire system. The trauma therapist carries out careful detective work, to get the answers to various questions. Which parts know about the memory? Which 'action systems' are they in? What is activated in the various emotional parts? Which ones are disturbed by the memory? Which of them should be present in the therapy room, and which should be excluded, when specific work is done?

Overcoming resistance

In the third phase of phase-oriented, trauma-focused psychotherapy, the patient's ability to stop avoiding intimacy is improved. Work on overcoming attachment and separation phobia is intensified. Here, the emphasis lies on integration and boosting the person's prospects of leading a workable, independent daily life.

Patients learn to overcome their resistance to change and difficulties in taking risks in a reasonably balanced manner. For the most severely traumatised, life has never rolled along with what we others would call normal smoothness. The patient's fear of a normal, secure life is sometimes a hard nut to crack.

Inner minefield

The section below describes very well how various parts of one and the same patient may perceive the relationship with their therapist during treatment. The description is taken directly from reality.

This man had an extremely violent history. He proved to have many different parts of the personality. Several of them had strong feelings, lived in the past and protected themselves in various ways. Some were at war with one another, and their inner dynamics were full of minefields. One of his raging, highly emotional parts of the personality, with control as its means of domination, said the following when he had made good progress in the treatment and stopped using violence:

'Yes, I was extremely angry with you at first. The problem was that I hadn't invited you... I kind of didn't know I was here in this body... You discovered me, and eventually I noticed I liked how you treated me... how you were towards me... You were kind... no one had ever been kind to me in particular...

'You opened your heart and you were like a friend... we sat here, just you and me, and you stepped into my heart and shared my pain... with me... and I like that, because no one ever felt what I do and understood how I feel. And that... made me human...

'All the kindness... all the compassion... understanding... I'd never got anything like that from anyone... I only got it from you... It made me change everything... how I look at myself... how I look at others and at the world... Everything changed and I was able to start listening to the other boys.'

This was an emotional part's experience. He thought the everyday part had initially forced him to go into therapy. This part had his own name, and his way of surviving had been fighting of one kind or another. He had long been imitating old perpetrators in his way of treating his body. Initially, he stayed in the background in relation to me, but acted violently against his own body between the therapy sessions — injuring himself by, for example, banging his head hard against the wall.

This emotional part of the personality was in fact reacting as he always had done. He was a fighter, and his habit was to resort immediately to violence as a defence. We (the therapist and the other parts of the personality) had to slow down and see what happened — invite and wait for him. He was noticed sitting watchfully in the background. Gradually, he calmed down and noticed that positive things were happening to the other parts. This discovery changed his approach. He initiated tentative contact attempts, tested me (TT) and finally arrived in the treatment room to work jointly with me.

What the hell happened?

This previously violent emotional part was, from the start, completely consumed by his own misery and sense of how badly he had been treated. At first, he had no space for any of the other parts' perceptions. He describes his state of mind as follows.

*'The boys didn't know about one another so... what you've done... and I don't know how you did it but... we started being able to share our thoughts... Before, I suddenly became a little boy and got stuck there, and when I came back, I wondered **what the hell happened?** When I finally started listening to the Little One and discovered what he'd been through, when I thought I'd been through the worst experience in life... then I suddenly became humble... If such a small boy could survive such things, then I can survive this. I thought.'*

The same part said: *'The treatment healed me... It made me whole and normal, because I used to think and just treated myself negatively and the criticism I had against myself was not really my own. Instead, every fingerprint, every rape, every blow and every assault I'd faced had left deep imprints on and in my body, and I thought people could see that on me... and you said they couldn't and those imprints weren't my fault... That made me so happy... so proud... and when you stop the self-criticism you start thinking positively... You no longer beat yourself up. Instead, I was able to show myself mercy, and doing that meant giving myself space.'*

Meeting of parts

One of the three everyday parts of the patient's personality later described his experience during the therapy.

'When I got the diagnosis and understood I was like bits and pieces of people, that there were teams and members and characters in me, it set me free. I became truly free — free from distraction, criticism, fear. Before, I just thought I was crazy...

'I got so free in that way that I discovered I had friends inside me. I could turn to them... and sort of explore my life... and get it into perspective... For me that's been the way with you... Every time you treated a boy inside me, you gave him therapy... it was different. It was different because they were different people... it made the boy feel better... it made him kind of come closer... get closer to me... in a way that made me feel whole... or, well... feel like one person.

'That was the main perspective, the challenge, and gave me the courage to keep coming here and making myself better, because if I'd never met you and if you hadn't made the boys meet, treated them and calmed them down... and got them to face their terror... like Peter, the little boy in me... To him you're the mother he never had, and that must be the core of someone like me being able to get better, have treatment and get well.'

Wordless speech

Much of our communication takes place without words. If we pay attention to trauma survivors' unconscious signals, we notice how clearly these convey what is going on within them. The body harbours much of our personal history. The body and mimicry tell of multilayered emotions. Psychotherapy methods developed by veterans such as Pat Ogden and Peter Levin focus intensively on the body.

Traumatised people usually have great difficulty to find a sense of safety in their own bodies. For a dissociating person, either the body is severely stressed and on the edge or it is disconnected and hard to sense at all. Often, involuntary movements occur. Trauma victims frequently have a protective, off-putting posture, indicating that they are prepared to defend themselves, or hide, at any moment. Sometimes, there is too much talking, and it is unduly forced, or traumatised people try to find words that elude them. Sentences are lost in a silent murmur. For a structurally dissociated person, it is important to find out which part of the personality is in charge. Who does the therapist need to reach out to right now? What possible tugs-of-war are taking place between different parts of the personality and how can I, as a therapist, support the patient?

All these common phenomena are important to notice and consider. Explicitly working in harmony with the body helps us to focus on the here and now in the therapy room. To make genuine healing occur, it is essential to include the body in the process. By putting the body at the centre, we can often bring recovery closer, but we must never forget also to take into account the desire of the various parts of the personality to control the body. We need to cooperate with them all.

To work and engage in a bottom-up as well as a top-down approach may be highly effective in treating both acute and severe chronic trauma. We are now seeing a great number of new studies that support us in our various body–mind approaches.

Focusing on the body

Not only patients communicate through their body language. The same applies to the therapists who treat them.

Therapists' ability to be present in their own body naturally affects their communication with patients. Embodying the compassion that we so sincerely wish to convey to traumatised survivors is central to the wordless communication in the therapy room.

At a lecture in Stockholm in September 2008, Professor Allan N. Schore talked about the need for psychotherapists to become observant and aware of their own bodies. He said that the depth and continuity of a psychotherapist's self-awareness strongly influences the depth of the exchange in a treatment process. If there is threatening material, this influence on the process is particularly important, since the psychotherapist's unspoken response to the patient's stories, which is immediately picked up by the patient, is even more important than the spoken words.

In Schore's view, if the patient has previously experienced threats, this will crop up again in the interface between patient and therapist. Can we trauma therapists allow ourselves to interact with the patient in the intimate space inside us? Dare we do so? Or is there a disconnection in us because we perceive the patient's moves, story and feelings as overwhelming or frightening? The patient's constant unspoken question is often: *Can anyone be with me when I'm with myself? If so, it's safe and secure, and I'm okay.*

Being with someone else, truly present, in the moments we share with patients can be challenging and difficult. Traumatised people have often developed the intuition to see potential danger in others. They observe the therapist's body language, wondering: *Is she afraid to hear my story? Does she really mean what she says? Can she be trusted? Is she really here for me? Is she present with me? Is there any risk at all that she is just observing me at a distance and thinking intellectually what she claims to stand for, or is the therapist really integrated in herself?*

These questions may not be deliberately conceived, but these issues are usually of burning importance to trauma survivors. Deficiencies can easily be interpreted as they have been explained so many times before. Their conclusions are negative: *I'm the one at fault; I'm so disgusting; I'm really not worth listening to*; or the like.

However, when we succeed in being truly present with the patients, it creates flexible scope to help them, based on what they convey that they need. For these deeply traumatised people, it does no good for a therapist to introduce a ready-made solution or concept. Instead, an opportunity for coexistence is created. This is revolutionary for a fellow human who has previously felt that other people are dangerous to be with. Silent, profound listening with no other agenda can be more healing than millions of words.

Can anyone love me?

In the therapist's role, we convey hope to a patient paralysed by hopelessness. Traumatised people can 'borrow' hope that they are not destroyed and emotionally broken. During the treatment, chances for the victims to notice the opportunities and joys of life can emerge. When self-trust begins to grow and patients recognise in themselves something that is good and possible to love, it creates what should always have existed: their ability to see how valuable they are.

We trauma therapists may all sometimes feel that we do not measure up. This is presumably inevitable. Is constant self-development perhaps our most important responsibility? After all, it will never be completed.

Both in my role as a therapist and as a private person, over and over again, I am hugely impressed by patients' healing capacity. Being part of this healing and seeing their triumph over trauma fills me with much joy, humility and gratitude.

Mind, consciousness and its nature

Despite research in the West and millennia of profound meditation in the East, no one can in fact explain in simple terms what the whole human 'mind' is. Nobody has found a place in us humans of which we can say *'This is our mind'* but 'that' is what constantly thinks in dualistic terms. In a cascade of thoughts and feelings, our mind automatically engages in valuation and projection in interaction with our environment. These thoughts and feelings are often very active and messy, pile up and give us neither space nor rest. We are often caught up in the content of all this, and the activity easily pushes us into feelings of dissatisfaction. Because of the constantly perceived threats, the mind of a traumatised person is often especially vigilant, in a single chaotic jumble of past and present experiences.

We can train our ability to avoid becoming quite so engrossed in our mind's intricacies. Then we create opportunities for glimpses of space between thoughts and feelings. When we learn how our mind works, we no longer need to blindly believe the content of all our thoughts. Although the feelings are hard to bear, we get help in noticing that they are constantly changing. Even the worst negative emotional storms are replaced by something else. Discovering this enables us to bear it when our thoughts and feelings are at their darkest, while knowing that some respite will come later.

When we practise quickly noticing what is happening inside us — observing when thoughts occur to us, noting what our bodily sensations are and what feelings arise — we can give ourselves some breathing space. Sometimes we have time to get signals at a conscious level. Then we can choose whether we want to act in response to that feeling, or just wait and endure what we are experiencing at that precise moment. Training the mind creates space to choose new ways to act, based on our real intentions. When we systematically practise awareness —through mindfulness exercises, for example — we train this ability and more.

There is a deeper dimension of our mind's nature, beyond the simple everyday way of being described above. It is something undistorted and original, an inner state of being in contact with something beyond thoughts, feelings, projections, values and the you–me or it–me division. We experience no 'wanting' or 'not wanting'. Instead, we perceive complete freedom from all such constructions.

Eastern meditation masters describe our mind as infinite. There is no limit to its capacity for alert awareness. They think this is the nature of our consciousness, but this deeper dimension is even more difficult to capture in words, grasp or explain.

Trained awareness: a key to health

We cannot help having the mind we have. The human brain and its interaction with the body and our surroundings function in a basic way that was shaped by evolution. Mental states organise the brain in different ways. Our thinking creates well-trodden trails and our attention tend to be swallowed up in these.

Although we lack control over the workings of our minds, as adults we are nonetheless responsible for how we *manage* our consciousness. We can practise creating distance from our thoughts and becoming flexible. This is an important key to health. We could all do with help in using this key, and if we have been affected by trauma, the locksmith and carpenter may naturally have to help.

Unfortunately, we are taught very little about how our senses and consciousness work. Rarely do children and young people in the West receive any instruction about how cunning our consciousness is. We are unaware of how it sets us difficult tests and easily creates loops of negative thoughts, or the fact that the human brain developed for several hundred thousand years and automatically fills thoughts, the content of which easily abducts us.

People in trauma-focused psychotherapy must work hard to put their past behind them, so that they can grow and flourish, despite the misfortune of suffering very difficult circumstances in life. About gradually being given a chance to practise his ability to become the captain of his own ship, one male patient said: *'At last, I can do something myself. I'm practising. Sometimes it works. Sometimes I'm totally lost, but it's a superb feeling to know a bit about what to practise.'*

East meets West

Internationally, over the past 30 years, we have seen a veritable explosion in scientific research. Contemplative neuroscience, cognitive science and psychology are examples of areas where interaction between body and mind is being studied.

Many brain researchers, such as Richard J. Davidson and the late Francisco J. Varela, have shown the amazing plasticity of the human brain. A ground-breaking exchange between East and West started in 1987, with the aim of creating dialogue and building bridges between modern western research and eastern wisdom in areas like meditation and other contemplative traditions.

Davidson and Varela were involved in the founding of the prestigious **Mind & Life Institute**, where research topics have included the first-person perspective in cognitive sciences. Many famous people in the western and Buddhist worlds alike have been, and still are, involved in the Institute's activities: His Holiness the 14th Dalai Lama, Adam Engle, Matthieu Ricard, Thupten Jinpa, Alan Wallace and the Venerable Amchok Rinpoche, to name a few. The Institute has now long ensured that dialogues, bridging conferences and research meetings are held.

Communication to date and under way in the body–mind field is extensive. We have tracked down a great deal of important knowledge, but much remains to be done. Perhaps we in the West should be especially careful. We have a habit of using scholarly or academic research results as if they were *whole* truths. There is always a risk of simple interpretations and over-generalisations. We are easily biased in favour of cognitive knowledge and tend to believe that it provides the whole picture, and that we know and understand more than we actually do.

In Buddhist psychology and philosophy, there is deep awareness that we cannot possess wisdom without practical work. We need to practise and observe our various states of consciousness so that we learn how they work. This practical training is essential. We cannot just learn theory and then understand. As the well-known Tibetan leader His Holiness the 17th Gyalwang Karmapa points out, according to a Tibetan proverb much intellectual work may result in many accumulated thoughts, but not in more wisdom.

A new and exciting project has recently been launched in Tuscany, Italy, and construction of the venue is due to start shortly. At the emergent Center for Contemplative and Scientific Research (CCR), meditation and science will meet. The CCR is to be led by Dr B. Alan Wallace, a world-renowned Buddhist scholar and teacher since the 1970s. The intention is, in collaboration with researchers from around the world, to address two closely related issues of human existence: What is the nature of genuine well-being? And what is the nature of human consciousness?

Awareness

Mindfulness, awareness, has been defined by the Zen Buddhist monk Thich Nhat Hanh as the practice of being fully present and alive, body and mind united, the energy that helps us to know what is going on in the present moment. Practising awareness with a traumatised person is a resource if it is done in a way adapted to the individual. I usually let patients record the personalised instruction so that they can practise at home too.

For traumatised people, perceptions of time and space often cause difficulties. Their experience does not tally with other people's. They may therefore benefit considerably from being guided in mindfulness training adapted to the individual. One important aspect of the training is *not judging* when our thoughts entangle us or we become absorbed by bodily sensations and feelings. Traumatised people are often quick — usually faster than others — to blame themselves. The training needs to be done gently and carefully. Sometimes we come across instructions and texts that teach mindfulness as 'being in the present' but omit the necessary aspect of practising non-judgement.

Honest with oneself

Practising awareness is an exercise in getting down into your own body and being mentally and physically unified. In people with dissociation, this unity is always lacking. The patient needs to practise listening inward, and asking: *What is it like to be in my body, here and now?* One of the most important aspects of the guidance is to practise honesty with oneself. The healing is based on honestly admitting to oneself what is happening in there. It is an exercise in being instead of doing. To enable complete honesty, the aspect of not judging must be part of the training.

The ability to 'descend into the body' can be trained in many ways. Instructions are varied and carefully adapted to the person. A well-functioning instruction, taken from meditation, is to 'put a little note' with a word on each thought or feeling that crops up. Research shows that this immediately and automatically reduces the reaction that appears in the amygdala. The intensity of a feeling diminishes as soon as it is described in individual words. If you want to increase the effect, you can create metaphors and use symbolic language. Best of all is usually when the therapist guides the patient to formulate metaphors and symbols that are emotionally charged for that particular person. Noticing thoughts or feelings in this way is a powerful method for easing the reaction.

Another step that may look easy to others is to practise making decisions. Decisions about quite small matters in everyday life also increase the individual's sense of control. For a person with many dissociative parts of the personality, the key is often making joint decisions. This may range from all the parts of the personality daring to stand up for their own wishes to coping with abandonment of their own approach and being ready to compromise. The training also creates a sense of satisfaction, which can be something of a pleasant surprise for the patient. At the same time, the decision-making becomes an exercise in thinking that one is doing something that may be regarded as good enough. This perception is hardly something a traumatised person can usually enjoy.

Training compassion

Compassion plays an important role in the treatment. Compassion is the feeling that arises when one is confronted with the suffering of others and feels motivated to relieve this suffering. While empathy refers more generally to our ability to adopt another person's perspective and experience someone else's feelings, compassion reflects a genuine will to relieve the other's burdens — wanting to help. Self-compassion is the ability to direct our compassion at our own person and, accordingly, within and among the parts of ourselves.

Neuroscience has succeeded in showing that pride is the most powerful feeling for activating the brain's reward system. Practising self-compassion creates opportunities for us to feel some pride, which makes us feel better. When we also practise noticing positive things that we are grateful for, this activates key parts of the brain that boost production of substances that make us happier.

In Germany, Professor Tania Singer has done research relating to neuroscience and compassion. She points out that not just the brain is involved. Plasticity and training potential also apply to our immune system, stress system and, not least, behaviour. Thus, we can develop our capacity for compassion.

Compassion, self-compassion and mindfulness have usually withered away in traumatised people. Full of tension inside, they are seldom in the habit of noticing these abilities. However, with the right training, their plasticity can be used positively. Provided that the training is adapted to the individual, it becomes a basis for development in mildly traumatised people, as well as in those with the most complex structural dissociation. Traumatised people should not have to be deprived of the joys of life. They too should have the chance to experience them.

Our hope is that this book will shed light on traumatised people's difficulties, opportunities and needs for the right treatment. Survivors and their relatives have much to gain from diagnosis and treatment becoming available and more effective. A little further on, we will look more closely at the financial benefits that accrue to us all when severely traumatised people receive the necessary treatment for trauma and dissociation.

But first you will meet Felicity.

SIXTH STORY

Felicity did not know what self-compassion was when she met TT. She was referred by a doctor who had realised that she was traumatised. Felicity was being tossed about, from one part of her personality to another, and felt very unwell. She had memory gaps and trusted no one — neither the parts inside herself nor other people around her. This was mixed with utter terror of trying to trust someone. Her inner conflict about who knew and should decide what to do was reflected in her attending or not attending the therapy, and talking about her experience or shutting down and trying to cope with it all by herself. It was a nonstop tug-of-war.

The City Court's verdict on her father's murder of her mother was a black-and-white document proving that Felicity had not just imagined everything. After a while, she took the document to TT and asked her to keep it until Felicity had advanced far enough in her recovery to be able to cope with the truth herself.

Christina Lejonöga : Annica Lilja Ljung

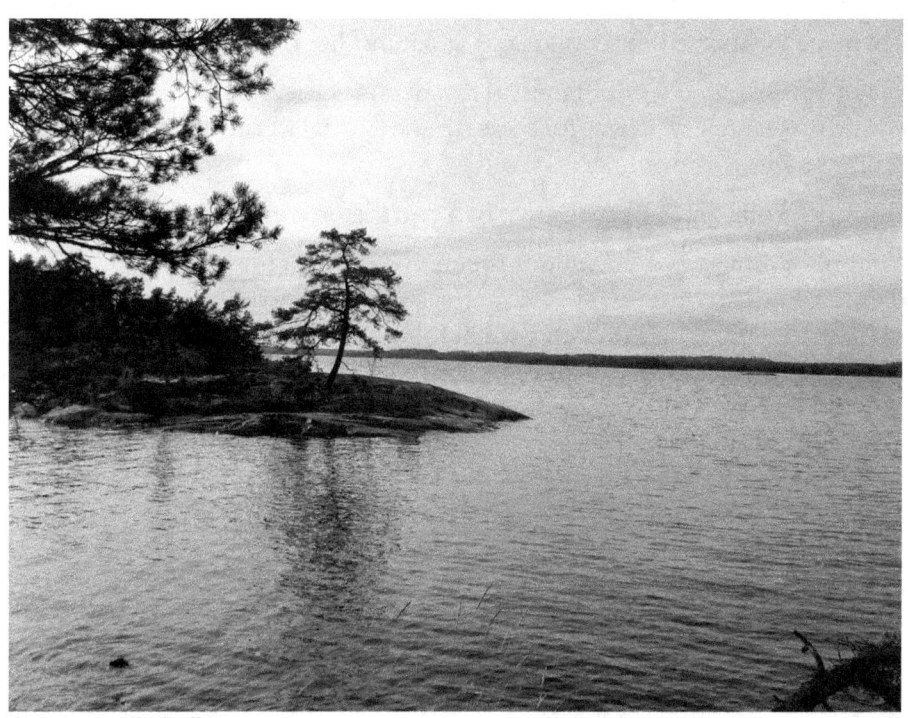

By Annica Lilja Ljung

Felicity

Felicity's father shot her mother to death and was committed to a high-security psychiatric unit. After two years in family homes, the children were taken from the security of their foster parents' care and placed with their father.

'I'm forced to live with my mother's murderer. It's a grim upbringing that drives me straight into the arms of a dangerous, destructive man. Reality is unbearable. No wonder I disappear into myself.'

My name's Felicity; I'm 39 years old and a mother of four.

My father migrated from France to Sweden in the 1960s, when Swedish companies were crying out for foreign labour. Over time, he married my mother and she moved here too.

First my brother was born. Barely two years later, I entered the world.

I'm only two when Mum realises the marriage was a mistake. She wants a divorce. She can't bear to stay in that destructive marriage, so she moves to Västerås, taking us children with her. Dad doesn't accept the divorce and begins persecuting my mother.

Alone in the universe

When I'm three years old, Mum meets a new man. Then Dad snaps. He charts Mum's life and works out a detailed plot to kill her. Before my five-year-old brother's eyes, Dad shoots both Mum and her new husband in the head. Both die on the spot. It's a sheer execution. My brother sees and hears everything. Afterwards, he says 'Dad BANG BANG.' Over and over again, my brother repeats 'Dad BANG BANG.'

Many hours later, I'm found in bed at home. Alone. Weeping. I remember none of it. Or rather, I have no conscious memories. But my body recalls the terror and sense of total abandonment. Maybe I was just left alone for a short while because I was sleeping. Perhaps Mum would come back soon?

But Mum never returns. The horrendous experience is stored in my body: I'm thirsty, hungry and scared, crying desperately. But no one comes and picks me up, consoles or reassures me. I'm alone in the universe, understanding nothing. Perhaps it feels as if I'm going to die, because that kind of feeling is etched deep inside me.

In the murderer's arms

My brother and I get placed with a foster family in Gävle, in the north of Sweden. We miss our mother but are safe and well off with the new family. I feel at home.

Dad is committed to a high-security psychiatric unit. After eight months there, he's already allowed to see his young children. We have to go to Beckomberga Hospital in Stockholm to visit him. Soon he begins to be granted unsupervised leave. It isn't long before Dad brings a new woman from France here and remarries.

When he becomes a free man, after two years, he demands custody of us. He threatens to take his own life if he doesn't get his children back, and he gets his way. Although we are so happy in our new family and despite our foster parents' intensive efforts to keep us, my brother and I have to move in with Dad and his new wife.

After two years' safety with our foster parents, the authorities decide we have to be separated from them and grow up with the man who murdered our mother. No one tells us that Dad has killed her. To this day, I don't really know what my brother remembers of what he saw: that Dad committed premeditated murder, shooting two people dead.

My brother and I are so young. We have no idea what awaits us.

Good girl

Dad is a workaholic, hard on himself and even harder on us. His new wife is very young, oppressed and ignorant about how to look after children. I sense that she doesn't care about me, and that she'll never be satisfied.

Dad works his way up and buys several restaurants. Increasingly, life revolves around money. The adults are always arguing about it. There is chaos at home. Dad is violent to my stepmother and she beats me, a small child. It scares me so much that I pee in my pants.

When I'm eight, my little brother is born. Then everything gets even worse. My elder brother and I are forced to work until late at night. Dad simply locks us into the restaurant. If we don't work properly, we have to go to bed hungry without supper. Our stomachs protest.

At school, I'm so tired that I hid in the loo to get some sleep. I lie down on the stone floor with my jacket as a pillow, close my eyes and disappear. I'm only eight or nine at the time.

All the same, I have to be good at schoolwork. To get Dad's approval, I have to score 100 per cent on the tests. That's the only time it feels good, when he says I'm clever. He's always on at me, giving me a terribly hard time, manipulating and pressuring me with his many demands.

Who can I trust?

Dad is powerful and manipulative, especially towards women. He has money and power. Dad's harsh and our stepmother even harsher. She punishes and hits me. I'm like her maid; I have to look after the household and my little siblings and work at the restaurant. We're like Cinderella and the wicked stepmother. All her relatives force me to scrub, clean and look after their children. My stepmother conveys the feeling that I really don't belong there, that I should be happy and grateful for living there and eating my fill. The sense of inferiority creeps in under my skin.

I'm forced to adapt. I have to be careful not to challenge my stepmother and make her angry. I get worn out, and carry great sadness inside me. I'm lonely, often worried and apprehensive. I daren't trust anyone an inch. Strangely, I see Dad as my saviour. True, he's mean too, but not as cruel as our stepmother. But Dad doesn't defend me. I'm totally defenceless.

To protect myself, I shut myself down and make myself tough. I screen off my emotions. Trying to take control of external reality, I start frenetically washing and wiping dry. I clean like a maniac. Scrubbing and sweeping becomes like a safe ritual.

Something wrong with me

The hard life continues. I adapt to what is expected of me. I work in the restaurant kitchen and, at home in the laundry room, wash towels and tablecloths from the restaurant. Nothing is voluntary in my life. Nothing is normal.

I grow up quickly. I'm not allowed to play, be with friends, have free time or just do nothing. That's just the way it is. I feel terribly ashamed. To prevent this from being revealed, I avoid other children. All the time, I think it's my own fault, that there's something wrong with me. *If I make a really big effort to be even nicer, more docile, more diligent and quieter, then maybe I'll be good enough and things will improve...*

My stepmother's anger rules. On a good day, I'm allowed to watch TV with my siblings. On a not-so-good day, I'm banished to the upper floor and forced to have supper alone.

My father's a womaniser, emotionally manipulative and violent towards the women in his life. My stepmother becomes bitter, cruel and greedy. She starts sending me to the shopping centre to steal dresses and makeup. For several years, I sneak into greenhouses and steal geraniums and other plants. *'You're a good thief,'* she praises me when I get home with the stolen stuff. As a child, what don't you do to have a decent life?

Without love, you thirst for affirmation. Of course I want to be obliging. Being 'good' and helpful gives me some value. When I steal for my stepmother, she's nice to me. She doesn't lock me into an upstairs room. I'm allowed to have supper with my younger siblings and feel normal for a couple of hours.

I know it's wrong to pinch flowers from people's private gardens, but I have to do it. When my stepmother is angry with Dad, she forces me to steal vouchers from his till at the restaurant. She's frustrated and takes it out on me. I daren't say no, or show my feelings.

Born out of wedlock

My brother and I look very like our mother. Every time Dad sees us, he's reminded of her. People wonder and ask: *'Who's the children's mother? Where is she? Why isn't she around?'*

Dad's emotionally closed towards us. Perhaps he's the same towards others. How else can he bear what he's done? I have no understanding of the context. Nor do I know the truth.

Somewhere inside me, I feel something isn't right. I know a secret is hidden in the family, but I have no idea what it's about. I just feel acutely uncomfortable.

For a long time, I think our stepmother is my real mother. When I'm eight or nine, I begin to sense that something was wrong. *Why don't I look like her at all? Why's my brother so sensitive? Why does he have such a strange relationship with Dad?*

I never get to hear what happened. It's covered up. But somehow, I gradually understand she isn't our real mother. I remember my brother's look: that he knew. I both know and don't know, as if I'm shielding myself from the truth. I keep a distance. I'm kind of not there.

Once when Dad's angry and about to beat my brother, I get between them. That arouses his rage. I'm told I'm a bastard and that Mum was a whore. Suddenly I realise: *my stepmother isn't my real mother.* I feel in my heart that I don't belong to them. That's a new jigsaw piece that's hurled at me.

My secret life

One day, when Dad and my stepmother have been arguing and she's furious with him, she points at him and shouts, *'There's your mother's killer!'* I hear her words, and they lodge deep in my mind, but everything feels very unreal. There's chaos inside me. Does she say such horrible things because she hates Dad? To make me hate him too? If what she says is really true, I'm terribly ashamed of my father. *What, did he murder my mother? No, surely not.* I can't take that in.

That sense of unreality and chaos is difficult to describe. What am I to believe? What's right and wrong? What's true? Like that thing about birthday presents. My little sister gets her own dog on her birthday. On my birthday, I get nothing — absolutely nothing. It's kind of obvious. The injustice is right there in front of my eyes, but I don't see it. The truth is too painful. I shut down, and live my own life inside my head. Because I don't belong there, I create the feeling of being in my own reality. My secret life.

Outwardly, Dad's a successful entrepreneur who runs several restaurants and makes plenty of money. We live in Täby, a wealthy suburb in north Stockholm. Dad has the neighbourhood's finest villa, and we can afford to go on holiday. But under the surface, I live in misery. My stepmother says straight out, *'You're not one of us.'* I feel I'm a burden. I have to be on my guard, ready to defend myself, all the time. I live in constant fear of the next attack.

Locked out

Dad's a krona multimillionaire. Outwardly, everything looks fine, but my brother and I live like slaves. While our younger siblings get fine new jeans, I have to pinch clothes out of the neighbourhood charity clothing bank. When I pull out the clothes, I feel desperately ashamed and sprint away, fearing that someone in my class will see me and I'll be teased.

I seek peace and security. To be free, I run away from home. The plan is to go to Stockholm's central underground station, T-Centralen, but I don't dare. I return home but am too afraid to go in, so I sit in the cold, dark woodshed, shivering. I know I've messed up but don't understand how I'll ever be able to go back into the warm house. I'm ten years old and infinitely alone.

Our stepmother and father take our younger siblings and travel to their newly bought house in France. My brother and I are left alone in Stockholm. For several weeks, we have to do our best to manage. We live on sliced bread, with only a toaster to cook with. I'm 12 years old. We're excluded from most of the house — a locked door keeps us out of the ground floor. We have access only to the upstairs part, and are unable to enter either the kitchen or the living room. Dad has locked us out of his home. Our home. He doesn't trust us.

I'm loyal. I go to school, work at the restaurant and behave myself.

All that is happening here in Sweden, in a safe, affluent Stockholm residential area, in the 1990s.

Cut off

I become increasingly aware that our family is different, and that the adults around me are very much out of line. I know what's expected of me. I become a specialist in adapting myself and, at the same time, living my own internal life. Every Saturday morning, I get up early to cook an omelette for Dad and prepare it just as he likes it. He says my omelettes are much tastier than my stepmother's. I lap up the praise.

At school, I feel like an outsider. Not like the others. I cut myself off from my classmates because I'm ashamed. I get used to the loneliness and convince myself I don't need any friends. *I'm special; I can manage fine without you.* That idea protects me and helps me accept my outsider status.

In the evenings, I cook at Dad's restaurant and have no time to do homework. At school, I'm almost always tired, but keep up appearances. I so desperately want to prove I'm good. That's my way of surviving — avoiding the feeling that I'm not good enough. I'm very tough on myself. The need to be good creates anxiety. Two hours before a history test, I desperately read the book about the Second World War, absorb the facts and then take the test. The result is good, but I soon forget it all.

Forbidden pleasure

One of my teachers lives next to Dad's restaurant. He goes there, drinks and boasts about how good I am. Dad gets very proud. Sometimes I feel some kind of bond with him, and it gives me a bit of security in the midst of the insecurity. I remember Dad's words: *'Felicity, you're a clever girl. You're like me! One day, you'll inherit everything.'* But he's manipulating me. Dad just sees my brother and me as labour, and wants to profit from us.

Sometimes I play truant from the last lesson of the day, and go into town and to the cinema. I need rest to have the energy to work in the kitchen all evening and until two o'clock in the morning. I find pleasure in the fantasy world of the movies. When I lose myself in a film, I get some freedom. Cutting myself off from reality feels good. Then I don't need any friends.

Years pass. No one reacts, except one of my teachers who tells me I work too much. She goes to my father's restaurant and talks to him, but it doesn't change anything.

Once, when my stepmother wants to send me to the restaurant although I'm very tired, I suddenly answer back. *'You bloody witch!'* I scream. Then she forces Dad to choose. *'It's me or your daughter,'* she threatens. The outcome is that I have to leave. Dad's betrayal is a heavy blow to me. I feel worthless.

I'm often hungry. At the restaurant, I'm not allowed to eat until I've finished working. My very strongest memory of hunger is associated with the smell of petrol and oil. Dad forces me and my brother to clean the garage. It feels like the job will take forever, but we aren't allowed out of the garage until we're finished. Never before have I been so hungry.

I don't really understand it myself, but I develop eating disorders. I need to be in complete control of everything before I allow myself to eat. I clean the whole house manically although my stomach is protesting and I feel sick.

Abused trust

Life goes on. I'm severely restricted. Going to a party or on a school trip is unthinkable. I'm so used to adults having power over me that I don't react when my uncle makes sexual advances. He's the only one in the family who's kind to me, and I like him a lot. Trust him. My uncle says *'Come on, Felicity!'* and lures me into going to a place where no one can see us. I'm completely caught off guard when he starts groping me.

It feels very strange when my uncle exposes himself to me in the restaurant kitchen and wants me to touch his body. It's so disgusting down there in the cellar. It smells acrid and mouldy, and rats scamper about. Undocumented immigrants who have to slave for meagre wages live in the storeroom.

My uncle takes the opportunity when no one else notices. I'm hungry for a bit of affection and I like him, but not what he does. Still, somehow it's worth it. I shut myself off. Afterwards, it feels like everything is my fault. I'm young and pretty, so I suppose I'm to blame.

The assaults begin when I'm 13 and go on for several years, in both Sweden and France. It feels good to get attention and affirmation and to feel special, but it happens in completely the wrong way. He abuses my trust. I know what he does to me and makes me do to him are wrong. Yet I don't understand what a betrayal of me it is. I don't think of telling anyone so as to get help in stopping it. I'm so much in the habit of being used and feeling ill at ease. That's how life has always been.

Out of the child prison

My uncle is the only one who dares criticise my father and stepmother — the only person who defends us and argues with Dad when he goes too far. My uncle bribes me with love. That's our secret. I'm scared, but don't want to lose him. The whole thing is confusing and unpleasant. Yet again, that feeling of unreality and chaos returns.

After a while, I try to tell a relative about the abuse, but I'm not believed. It's immediately hushed up. Knowing it's wicked to betray a secret, I feel even more ashamed. Eventually, I start to distrust myself. *Am I dreaming? Have I imagined everything?* But no, I know all the sick stuff I'm subjected to is true.

Dad knows how to get power over people. Suddenly I'm getting 50 kronor a day when I work at the restaurant. My life feels meaningful. I save every krona I earn. I hide the money under a stone, and dream of getting out of my child prison. Finally, I'm able to travel to my grandmother in France. I love the people in the countryside and the unspoilt natural surroundings in the mountains. I feel free there and find something I miss in my life.

Desperation

After the summer, the slavery at home in Sweden restarts. Somewhere inside me, I begin to understand that life shouldn't be like this. It isn't right. Finally, we've had enough, my brother and I. When I'm 15, we start planning to murder our father. One of Dad's employees promises to help us. He's heartily sick of peeling potatoes for 100 kronor a day in the damp cellar, and tired of Dad's greed and dictatorial ways. We travel around Stockholm's underworld looking for a firearm. The plan is never put into action, but our genuine desire to kill our father shows how desperate we are.

The situation is untenable. I'm exhausted. My brother and I run away. We simply can't bear to stay in Dad's power. We stay away for several weeks. Nicolas, a young Frenchman, helps me. We meet in the Metro and get talking. He shows me to an apartment where I can hide.

Dad gets the police involved. When the hiding place is revealed, I become desperate and hang by my hands from the balcony so they won't get hold of me. But I can't get away. I'm forced to slither down the drainpipe, and cut my leg on the sharp metal.

Before I get into the police car, Dad whispers in my ear: *'Don't tell them anything. Reveal nothing.'* For the first time ever, I get confirmation that the sick things I've experienced are true. Dad's scared.

Slain

The escape means that I'm placed in a residential assessment unit, among burglars and prostitutes. There, the staff have no idea what my problem is. I have no drug problems. I don't walk the streets. I'm well-behaved and diligent.

That summer at the assessment unit is the best part of my childhood. Never have I felt so well. It's like staying in a hotel and being on holiday. At last I can breathe. I run in the forest, play football and tennis, go bowling and bathing. Running is wonderful. My 'contact person' says I'm a natural and registers me for a race. I do well — as always.

During my childhood, I don't know for sure that my father killed my mother. All I know is that Mum died when I was little and is buried in the Skogskyrkogården cemetery. That incident when I was 12, and my stepmother's claim that Dad had murdered Mum, have been wrapped up somewhere deep inside me, and have disappeared. Now I start investigating what really happened when I was little.

My contact person helps me. Together, we go to the cemetery to look for Mum's grave. I'm full of expectations as we walk around the gravestones, searching. When we find the spot, I get a shock. There's just a plastic tag with a number. It feels desolate.

In the church records, we read 'No relatives' and 'Slain' How can it say that? That isn't true! The shock is total. I feel I'm falling apart.

Afterwards, the guilt settles like a stone in my stomach. I know I've done something that's absolutely forbidden. I remember my stepmother's words: *'Don't dig into that. You'll put us to shame. It's not your dad's fault that she died. She was unfaithful left, right and centre and had herself to blame. Forget she ever existed.'*

Part of me is ashamed of defying the ban. Another part is proud of my liberation. It's my right to know the truth about my parents.

Lip service

Thanks to my contact person, I get confirmation that Dad shot Mum dead and was committed to a high-security psychiatric unit. That I've grown up with a killer. We talk about how badly my stepmother and her relatives have treated me, and I tell her about my uncle. I put my traumatic experiences into words.

After the social investigation, I go to a new foster home — this time in Skåne, in the south of Sweden. There, the idea is for me to be a lodger and look after myself. Everyone thinks I'm so mature for my age, but I feel I've gone astray in life. I accuse myself. How could I let Dad down like that? After the second day in the home, I take the train back to Stockholm to live with him. I feel a strong emotional dependence. He's my father, after all.

But I don't stay there. Dad makes me think everything bad that has happened is caused by his wife. I want to get away from my stepmother and Sweden, so he sends me to France. For four months, I live with my paternal aunt in a country where I was neither born nor grew up. It gives me a sense of security to get up early in the morning and milk the cows with Gran, but Grandpa is cruel. Just like Dad, he loves money and power. I don't feel good at all.

In Sweden, Dad resolutely continues to run his restaurants. After returning from France, I have to work hard. Escape is impossible. Going to upper secondary school isn't an option. Loyally, I work for Dad. Aged 16, I shoulder responsibility for opening and closing the restaurant for the day. Dad convinces me that one day I'll inherit his empire. *'Everything will be yours, Felicity,'* he promises. *Okay,* I think, *I'm not getting an education and I can't hang out with friends or guys, but I'm going to be rich.*

Our home — a crime scene

Two months after returning home, along comes a major new disaster in my life. Daily life is characterised by constant intrigues and arguments between my stepmother and father. The stay in the high-security psychiatric unit hasn't cured Dad's violent side. When he learns that my stepmother has met another man, he goes completely crazy with jealousy. He himself does what he wants with women, but when his wife meets someone he sees red.

Dad closes the restaurant and goes home. My younger brother and I are with friends in Skärholmen, a suburb south of Stockholm. The anxiety gnaws at my stomach. I sense that something is going on and call home to check the situation. My stepmother says in a scared voice, *'You've got to come home, Felicity. Your Dad's threatening me.'* I hear Dad's voice in the background, sounding very strange. Quickly, I head home. I hold my little brother's hand and we half-run all the way from the bus. When we get home, I instantly realise something was wrong. The door is open. I get worried in earnest, and tell my brother to stay outside and wait there.

I rush in and see bloody marks on the floor. My stepmother, the mother of my little brother, is lying in the hall, in a pool of blood. Dad has stabbed her. I see the blood pumping out of a deep wound in her throat.

Almost unconscious and with her eyes rolling, she's breathing very strangely. I realise this is really bad. I leap into action, emotionally sealed off. I try to stop the blood, which is gushing out rhythmically. I make an emergency call and then discover that my brother has come in and is staring in shock at his mother.

He's nine years old. I take him by the hand and we flee from there. Dad has left, taking with him our sister, a small girl of only four. I leave my brother with a friend and search desperately for my elder brother. I know who he usually hangs out with and I simply have to get hold of him. I have nowhere else to go. But I can't find him.

Our stepmother survives the attack. Dad is detained for the stabbing. Our home is cordoned off for a crime scene investigation. I can't be there, so I keep away and sleep in stairwells. I'm so awfully ashamed of our family and the horrendous things Dad has done. Afterwards, I just remember fragments of that period. Somehow, my brain shuts off the terrible things that have happened.

Free at last

Dad's in police custody. My stepmother's in hospital. I feel very much alone. Finally, I contact the Social Services, and they arrange for a place in a temporary hostel for young people. My only thought is to try to keep the business going, so I loyally go on working at Dad's restaurant. But on the phone, Dad tells me I now have to look after myself, and that I should get a family of my own.

Life feels unbearable. I want to get away. I leave Sweden and travel back to France to meet Nicolas, the guy who helped me when I was on the run back home in Stockholm. Nicolas was born in Egypt but grew up in France. I trust him. He's my way out of childhood's tight grip. I'm free at last.

Nicolas is very fond of me. It feels so nice that someone is taking care of me and wants me. I'm not in love, but need security. I thirst for love and affirmation. I want to start a family. That desire is strong, perhaps because my own family has split up, or maybe because I want to show Dad my life is a success. Dad still has a strong mental hold on me. I'm 17 years old and extremely insecure.

After my 18th birthday, we get married. Now I'm proud. My stepmother has often told Dad, *'Your daughter will be a whore and get pregnant without being married.'* It feels good to be able to retaliate and prove her wrong.

It soon turns out that I've got out of one hell and into another that's even worse. Nicolas drinks a lot and is very jealous. If another man looks at me, I get my ears boxed. He yells at me, *'It was you! You! You! Admit it was you who flirted with him!'*

I find I'm suddenly living a life under constant surveillance. Isolated. Controlled. I'm never, ever allowed out alone. But I'm used to being a victim. The odd blow doesn't matter. I'm hardened and feel nothing.

Cracked ribs

Nicolas tends to feel inferior easily. I see that he feels bad and I'm sorry for him. When he knocks down drinks or pills, he takes it out on me, his mother or his sister. Afterwards, he's remorseful, knowing that he's done wrong. Over and over again, I forgive him. I do it numerous times, in the hope that there'll never be a next time or that another solution will turn up. I cling to my husband, the perpetrator — the only security I have. I seek closeness at all costs despite the danger. Part of me believes it's the only way.

I have to do my best and I live like a slave, just like when I was a child. I get up early in the morning and wash the family's laundry by hand, cook, clean the whole house and take care of his old grandmother. At mealtimes, I'm not allowed to join them and sit at the table. I don't count as a family member. I'm only a servant, just as I've been used to in the past. It feels normal. Insight comes too late: I, who have lived with a dictator all these years, have thrown myself straight into the arms of another.

I feel obliged to have sex with him. I go along with what he wants. That's just the way it is. Maybe adapting is what my survival instinct tells me to do. Afterwards, it feels unreal. Was it rape or a reluctant sex act? The boundaries are moved and the coercion is normalised. In my inner chaos, pretty much everything is mixed up. All I know is what it's like living under coercion of various kinds. I can't see clearly.

Before long I get pregnant. My tummy swells and I'm very scared. Nicolas shreds my Swedish passport and breaks me down mentally. Soon he's half-killing me. Black eyes and cracked ribs are everyday incidents. I shut down and feel nothing. It's like not being there when it happens.

Nicolas isn't himself when he beats me. He's ice-cold, and under the influence of alcohol and drugs. I can't get through to him. Several times, I think he's going to kill me — that I really will die. Even his own mother is terrified of him. Once, when Nicolas is broke and she doesn't give him any money, he smashes half the house.

It's disappointing. I feel sad, ashamed and helpless. Going home to Sweden is unthinkable. I have nothing to return to there. I don't want my sadistic stepmother and her family to see that I've failed. I have to get through it all, whatever the cost.

Wanted

Throughout my life, I've been incredibly hard on myself. I've driven myself on manically. I've adapted to extreme conditions, shut down my feelings and worked energetically to succeed in shutting out all the unbearable things. That's been devastating. I'm continuing in the same way, but without understanding what I'm doing: I don't see the repetition and have forgotten a lot. I find excuses for Nicolas's actions. I close my eyes to avoid seeing how wrong everything is, and his offences. I'm living far from home with a mentally disturbed man. He's exactly like my father, but much more violent. And now I'm expecting his child.

To find some peace, I begin to pray. I turn inwards and pray to God that my husband won't come home. That the nightmare will end.

Nicolas is a criminal — something I've had no idea about before. He's wanted for robbing people. Everything has got out of hand. We have to get away, but have no money. No matter how much I try to figure out how to do it, I see no chances of escaping on my own. I'm terrified.

I go to the Swedish Consulate and appeal for help. The woman understands that I'm in a bad way, arranges a temporary passport and supports me. After my mother's death I was awarded a large sum of money, but it was blocked until my coming of age. Now I need to get the money released. Unfortunately, it turns out that Dad has falsified my signature during his parole and stolen almost 100,000 kronor. He has not only taken my mother's life; he's also taken the compensation I was given after her death. Thankfully, there's enough money for tickets home.

Carton of milk

We manage to reach Sweden and get temporary accommodation in the city of Södertälje. That's when the real hell begins. Nicolas is on cocaine, and forces me to steal. He's violent and knocks me about so badly that I can't see. Severely injured, I'm taken to hospital and, from there, transferred to a women's shelter.

I'm extremely sad and feel dreadful. I don't know how I can help myself. Nicolas begs me to return to him from the shelter. His kind, warm, considerate and soft sides come to the fore. He talks about how he's going to change. He promises everything will be different. Nicolas is incredibly manipulative, and I let myself be persuaded. I forgive him. I so much want everything to be fine. For us to be a family — him, me and the baby.

But Nicolas is insanely jealous. He says he owns me. That I'll never get rid of him. When I try to escape, he laughs scornfully and says, *'Where will you go? You've got nothing to return to.'* I know he's right. I have nowhere to turn. He has the upper hand and I'm totally dependent on him. Exposed to his violence, I feel in his power, caught in his net. I don't even dare go shopping without him.

The abuse continues. His gaze is blank; his blue eyes are expressionless. He beats me so badly that the labour pains start. Already, in the seventh month, our little son is born. He weighs only as much as a carton of milk, and has to be in an incubator for two months. I feel nothing. No happiness. No fear.

I'm 19 years old, beaten by my husband, a new mother and completely shut down emotionally. Everything's a monotone inside me. Over and over again, I pray to God: *'Take this man out of my life.'*

Our son, Matteo, is discharged from hospital. I live in terror that Nicolas will shoot me. Why? After all, Dad shot Mum to death when he was really, really angry. A voice inside me says the same thing will happen to me. Daily life seems unreal and I feel no love for my child.

Boundless

Nicolas steals wallets at the pub, and forces me to go to shops and put goods in the pram. In the past, my stepmother forced me to steal. Now my husband is doing the same thing. I don't put my foot down and say no. I become the perpetrator's loyal helper, pretending nothing is happening and lying to myself. I'm a thief — and that's completely normal.

Several times, I report my husband for assault. I want to protect my child and myself, but withdraw the report every time, not daring to go through with it. I fail to protect myself, to defend my own boundaries. The violence has become normal in my life. It's as if I've become a different person from the real Felicity. So broken. So weak.

The abuse continues. My body aches and is sore. With cracked ribs, breathing is painful. My heart is heavy, like a stone. It's like being cut off. Isolated. The world is going on somewhere else. Finally, I end up at the women's shelter. Then a miracle happens in my life. Nicolas gets caught, goes to prison and is sentenced to expulsion. After a while, he is deported from Sweden to Egypt, the country of his birth. At last, I'm strong enough to take the decision to divorce.

But my self-esteem is at rock bottom. I feel broken down mentally. Even when Nicolas is gone, I feel I'm under surveillance. Life is perilous. It takes several months before I dare to go out alone. After all, he knows people everywhere...

A normal life?

Confused and easily scared, I lack resistance to my husband's manipulative power. When Matteo's a year old, Nicolas persuades me to travel to France and leave our son there with his relatives. As usual, Nicolas uses my past against me, saying, *'Don't ruin things for Matteo now. Give him a chance to feel loved and get attention. Leave him with my mother, who has time for him.'* Being psychologically dependent on Nicolas, I buy his reasoning and think our son will benefit from his grandmother's love.

In the past, I've done what my father told me to do. Now I'm obeying my son's father. I leave Matteo with his grandmother in France, go back to Stockholm and work. I earn money. I think everything will work out. I've worked my whole life, so I'm used to doing my duty. Somehow, I perceive a kind of freedom in that.

I work all summer. Then hope returns. Nicolas persuades me to help him one last time. If I show willing by getting him a false passport, flying to join him with it and accompanying him through passport control into Germany, he promises to leave me in peace in the future. Forever. *Might I finally achieve a calmer life? A normal life? Could I, perhaps, get away from being constantly terrified if I make this last contribution?* With that hope, I choose to believe Nicolas. I arrange a passport and join him in Egypt.

Desperation

When we meet, he's nice and cheerful. Together we fly to Berlin and manage to get past the passport police. Now Nicolas is in Europe again. I've kept my promise and am waiting for him to fulfil his part of the agreement and finally let go of me. Soon I'll get my son back and have a quiet life. He's going to let me fly on to Sweden.

But I don't get my freedom. Nicolas breaks his promise, takes me to a hotel and locks me in the room. He gets drunk and becomes transformed. Laughing scornfully at me, he says, *'Did you really think I'd set you free?'* He beats me up so badly that I get a crack in my cheekbone and bleeding in one eye.

Nicolas beats me black and blue. My eye swells up so I can't see. In desperation, I jump from the third-floor balcony. All I've got in my head is a desperate thought that I must free myself from my tormentor. I break my leg in the fall. People on the street help me, and I'm taken to hospital. There, a police officer watches over me. After the hospital stay in Germany, the Swedish Embassy helps me to return to Sweden.

Kidnapping

My son's still in France. I miss him a lot, but Matteo's father is there and won't let him go. Nicolas subjects me to emotional blackmail. On the phone, he says *'If you want your child, you'll have to take me too.'* Never! I want nothing to do with him, the man who hurt me so badly. I hang up. It feels like I'm dying inside. How will I get my son back without exposing us to daily danger, living with his father? I hope the relatives are kind to him, but I know so little about his life with them. It almost drives me crazy.

For two years, I have no contact at all with my son. To survive, I try to forget him. I feel shredded emotionally. I can't sleep. I feel terrible, and go in and out of mental hospital. I can't cope with work and shut myself in at home, watching one film after another to escape from my reality. Life is hopeless. Indifferent. I'm dreadfully disappointed with myself and feel like a very bad person.

In the end, my friends react, saying, *'You've got to get your child home.'* I get help contacting my municipality, which promises to pay for my trip to France. I'm granted sole custody of Matteo and the Swedish police force issues a temporary passport for him. Risking my life, I go to France. I'm 23 years old and lost in the world. My sole focus is on bringing him home to Sweden.

I manage to collect Matteo from pre-school. Although he hasn't seen me for two years, he knows I'm his mother. He's forgotten his Swedish, but recognises me and feels no fear. I take him in my arms, run for my life and jump into a taxi. I succeed in smuggling him out. It feels like kidnapping my own child. I don't feel good at all.

Overwhelming truth

At last I have my son with me again. But it isn't easy. Matteo is three years old and I understand now how he's suffered. He's been beaten a lot and is in a sorry state. I have to build everything from scratch. It's incredibly hard.

A few years go by. To earn money, I have several jobs in parallel. Throughout my life, I've worked too much and too hard. That's the only affirmation and encouragement I've ever received. *'You're so diligent, Felicity!'* people used to say. That's how I got my identity. Constantly, I had to learn to exceed my own limits, and push myself hard.

Now I'm continuing with the same pattern and being extremely strict with myself. At the same time, I'm terribly sensitive, reading other people directly — as I had to read my father and stepmother, to survive. I'm hardened, yet hypersensitive. Always feeling so much is a strain.

I brood over what really happened when Mum died, and where her family — my maternal grandparents, uncles and aunts — are. An enterprising part of me manages to get hold of the verdict document from Stockholm City Court, where Dad was convicted of murder. I also examine the preliminary investigation carried out by the police in Västerås. It confirms that the execution was planned.

Filled with burning anger and despair, I seek out Dad at work and shout, *'You bastard!'* at him. He's totally bewildered. *'The least you can do is to tell me where my mother's family is,'* I yell. He tells me.

So then I know, but I don't have the strength to act. Not yet. The thick pile of papers goes into the bottom drawer. I push the whole business away. The truth is overwhelming.

Betrayed

My son and I are extremely lonely, and I'm an incredibly tired mother. It feels like I'm far from measuring up, and I'm ashamed not to be strong enough to cope with my child. Matteo's now five, and talks a lot about his father. When they speak on the phone, Matteo's happy. Nicolas now sounds completely different. He says he regrets what he did when he was young and stupid. He apologises to me. He praises me, saying I'm the world's best mother. I very much want to believe him.

He launches an intensive persuasion campaign. Eventually, I'm unable to resist, and agree to our son being with his father over the summer. Matteo misses his father so enormously, and I find not letting them get together too difficult. So I take Matteo to France and we spend a week together there so that I can check how everything is going. Matteo is overjoyed. The hatchet is buried. Nicolas and I agree that our son will return to Sweden after the holiday. I have sole custody and am entitled to bring him home. In my fantasy world, I'm relying on that.

During the month, I work and get some rest from all the responsibility. In August, I send the airline ticket as promised. Expectantly, I wait at Stockholm Arlanda Airport — but in vain. Matteo doesn't arrive. My heart is constricted. His father has hidden him away abroad. Once again, I've lost my child.

How could I be so stupid and believed Nicolas? I know he's a liar! I feel guilty and can't forgive myself for putting my son and me in such an awful situation.

The shame and anxiety are horrendous. I accuse myself, asking *How could I do it, over and over again? What have I done to my son?* I begin to feel guilty about everything bad that's happened in my life. I feel I have myself to blame. An inner voice says I truly deserved all the terrible things other people have done to me. And I promise myself never to believe in Nicolas again. Otherwise, I'll never be free.

Chaos and death anxiety

In a desperate attempt to keep my feelings at bay, I throw myself into work. It's like being in a bubble. My head is completely in charge and I shut down my body, heart and feelings. I push myself harder than others. I rush around faster and faster to hold back the volcano of feelings and prevent an eruption. At home, I clean obsessively. In the evening, I — who have never been a drinker before — hit the bottle until I vomit. It's extremely self-destructive.

At the same time, I'm highly sensitive. I can neither eat nor sleep. Everything catches up with me, and I break down. I'm no longer capable of being strong. After years of fear and violence, it's all quite simply too much. My son's stuck with my husband's relatives, far from home. My life is falling apart like a house of cards. Reality feels fragmented and I suffer from severe memory gaps. People seem to be able to see straight into me.

In the evenings, I walk up and down the streets and am totally out of it. I hear inner voices that scare me. They say, *'If I go one way, there'll be one disaster, but if I go the other way there'll be another.'* There's no escape. Death anxiety takes over. I see my own funeral in my mind's eye. Everything feels unreal. I'm plunged into powerful flashbacks. Or am I going mad?

It feels like I'm no longer strong enough to exist. I get an impulse to step into the car and drive straight out onto the motorway. *'Crash, and then you'll escape everything!'* shouts the inner voice. But something keeps me alive. Matteo mustn't be subjected to what I went through. He mustn't lose his mum. He mustn't lose his mum. He mustn't lose his mum.

Into the fog

My anxiety doesn't let up. My heart beats hard in my chest and I can barely breathe. It feels like I'm not getting any oxygen at all into my lungs. I'm overflowing with unresolved despair. All hell is breaking loose. All reason is cast aside. Complete chaos rules inside me.

Finally, I collapse and end up in a mental hospital. After spending a few days there I'm sent home again, but feel worse and worse. I slide into a deep depression and escape into the darkness by swallowing a packet of antidepressant pills. Freed from the nightmare, I fall into the deepest of sleeps.

My life hangs by a fragile thread, but I have a guardian angel. Afterwards, I remember nothing. My sense of time has completely gone. I'm told I've been in a coma for three days. The hospital feels like a prison. I'm admitted to a psychiatric clinic and everything feels foggy from all the medication. My only goal is to get out of there.

For a year, I'm in and out of mental hospital. Several times, I try to take my life. I'm cast back and forth from anger to despair and resignation. Over time, there are various diagnoses: burnout, borderline, depression, schizophrenia, ADHD, bipolar… The care I receive is absolutely useless.

Eventually, the Social Services help me to make a fresh start. They pay the rent and other expenses like that. But no one checks up on how I'm feeling — or whether I'm keeping medical appointments or managing to look after myself. Reality feels fragmented. I neither eat nor sleep. I'm not up to managing my finances. My debts grow and still hound me to this day.

I'm treated in psychiatric outpatient care. The supportive counselling is of little benefit. At the same time, I attempt occupational training. Never, ever have I been given so much medication. I keep seeing new doctors. It feels like a merry-go-round. I feel challenged. *'Why can't you work?'* they ask. I don't have the strength to tell them how I feel deep down inside, to describe what I've been through. I feel I'm under suspicion — as if they just see me as a lazy immigrant.

Second chance

I'm broken down and damaged. I miss my son so much that my chest aches. I can't cope with seeing other children. Somehow, life goes on anyway. But my son's living in poverty and deprivation, and it feels like I'm allowing that. I've abandoned him, after all. During this time, I have no contact with Matteo, but send money to France for him to improve his situation. I feel guilty and want to compensate for letting him down. But his father spends the money on drugs. I slide into yet another period of illness. The doctors say it's a psychosis. In retrospect, I don't know for sure whether it was.

When I'm helped to sleep late for a few days, the anguish gradually lets go of me. Slowly, I move on to a reasonably normal life.

One evening when I'm in a restaurant with some girlfriends, we're served by a nice man. We get on well and, over time, become friends. Marcel's calm and respectful, and cares about me in a healthy way. I feel I can trust him quite well. That's a big thing for me.

For a long time, we're just friends. In time, we become a couple. My biological clock is ticking and soon I get pregnant. Aged 27, I give birth to my second child, a beloved daughter. It feels like I've got a second chance in life. I read all the books on child psychology and upbringing thoroughly. *Now I'll get everything right!*

Marcel helps me write a letter to Matteo's father. I'm no longer afraid of Nicolas. I have Marcel's support and he manages to resolve the deadlock. That's a big turning point in my life. Then the baby's born. Never before have I been so happy. Floating in my euphoric bubble, I decide to do my absolute best for my children.

The past comes knocking

When the baby's six months old, Matteo finally comes to Sweden with his father. Matteo is to stay with us. He's eight years old. We have a lot of catching-up to do. The first few months are very difficult for us. Matteo speaks no Swedish and it's obvious to us that his upbringing, during the years after being kidnapped by his father, has been extremely hard. Now I want to get everything right, and patch up everything that's broken. I do that well, but I don't *feel* well. I'm suffering from severe stress and shut down my feelings.

After just three months in Sweden, Nicolas gets arrested for robbery and is sentenced to nine months' imprisonment and expulsion from Sweden. He appeals the expulsion, on the grounds that he has such a good relationship with his son. Thank goodness I'm able to testify and describe all the troubles there have been. I've sacrificed so much in my life for that man. It's nice to see him sitting there in the dock, being held to account.

Since then, Matteo has lived with us. I get pregnant again, and soon our second daughter is born — my third child. That's a great joy. I struggle to live as ordinary a life as possible. Life is about my children being in a good situation. Of course, I want to give them everything I've never had myself.

Now I have to get everything right... but still, I don't feel at all well. I'm plagued by nightmares and repeatedly overpowered by flashbacks that cast me back to vile events I've experienced. I may be queuing at the till in the grocery store, with the push-chair and tired kids, when I suddenly start sweating and my heart starts pounding. The panic surges over me and I have a blackout.

Guilt and shame

To keep the anxiety away, I constantly do things with my children. I keep busy, and avoid feeling. That's my need for control. Throughout my life, I've struggled to be good enough. Battled to avoid feeling what those who had power over me were doing to me: Dad, my stepmother, Grandpa, my uncle and my first husband. Now I'm doing the same thing, repeating the old pattern to avoid feeling.

I never dare relax. When I've put the children to bed in the evening, I go to work and work all night. In the morning, I come home, wake up the kids, get breakfast ready, clean, go shopping and cook. I try to be perfect.

There's a voice inside me driving me to work hard so that I survive mentally. I have to endure, and shut down, to avoid feeling how sad I am. I have to adapt myself and be obliging, show myself to be good and invulnerable — just like to Dad and my stepmother. Otherwise, I'm invaded by shame and guilt.

But shut-down feelings don't die. They're encapsulated deep inside me and drain my energy. Under the surface they lie smouldering, burning away at me and triggering what seem to be odd emotional reactions in everyday life. The situation is unsustainable. I'm overcome by fatigue and lose all strength. I have nightmares that something terrible will happen. A loud alarm is going off inside me, and I can't escape from it.

Dissoci... what?

Finally, I meet a psychiatrist who understands I'm burdened by deep trauma. At last someone is listening, and the fact of my problems being linked to my childhood is being affirmed. *'You definitely shouldn't be here. You're in the wrong place,'* he says, and refers me for psychotherapy.

There, I meet TT. She finds that I'm suffering from post-traumatic stress, PTSD, and a dissociative disorder. I don't know what it is and don't even know there is anything called that. I go home and Google it online, and decide to give the therapy a shot.

Part of me is screaming for help. Another part just wants to be left alone and has her hands full with life's practical problems: how to cope financially and with the children. I gradually become slightly more stable, but it takes time. When TT starts to poke around in my soul, one part wants to tell my story, while I switch another off and warn her that it's dangerous to come close. One part of me thinks: *Oh my God, this is even worse than in mental hospital!*

Sometimes, in my sessions with TT, my stomach almost turns over. I get palpitations and want to get away. Sometimes I phone to cancel. Still, I keep on going there. At times it's a great relief to be able to describe what I've been through. A little hope is awakened.

Away from time and space

The papers about the preliminary police investigation and the City Court's verdict are still in my bottom drawer. Now the time's ripe: I'm ready to take in the truth. I go to TT with the verdict record in my hand. *'I want to know!'* Together, we read the thick pile of papers, and what I already knew is confirmed. I get terribly angry. I'm overwhelmed with rage that Dad murdered Mum... that the government agencies made me grow up with Mum's murderer... that I've been completely fooled. Yes, I'm desperately angry about everything and with everyone! TT says she'll keep the verdict record safe. Somehow, that makes me feel a bit freer and more secure.

I'm angry, but not sad. Elated, more like. At last I have vital keys for unlocking my story and life. In the documents are particulars of my mother's full name and birthplace. I feel a strong urge to find her relatives. If I'd gone on living with that verdict record in the drawer, deep healing would hardly have been possible for me.

Through therapy, I slowly begin to understand myself. I feel that I've sometimes lost touch with reality. The memory gaps have made me think I'm becoming demented — it'd that bad. Now I learn it's a matter of dissociation. When I kind of disappear into my head, away from the here and now, and from the sensations of time and space, I know it: *Oh here we go, I'm dissociating!* The reality around me feels fragmented.

Inside, I'm overflowing with recollections from the past. Although I've been out of touch with those memories, the child's experiences are merging with things that have happened to me as an adult. Then I behave like a terrified little child.

Sometimes I think all those awful things have never really happened — that they've just gone on inside my head. At the same time, I know too well that it's true. In the therapy, I learn that dissociation is a way for the body and brain to protect themselves. A way to survive a reality that brings too much pain.

Me against the world

Reluctantly, I realise my brain has divided me into several different parts of my personality, such as the scared child, the angry one, the sad one, the judgemental one, the hard-driving one and the vindictive one who wants to get her own back. *Shit!* I felt. *That's right!* That feeling of 'me and them'. Finally, the pieces fall into place in the puzzle that I've never managed to solve. Yet I feel a strong resistance. I don't want to hear about that. It hurts too much. The curtain goes down.

It takes two years to fully accept the idea. I'm living in denial. I don't trust anyone, not even my therapist. A strong part of me simply refuses to listen. She takes over and makes the decisions. I instantly switch to the denying part of my personality. It switches on and off without me being able to control what's happening. Still, I usually manage to go to the therapy. TT parries my remarks and helps me, giving me the strength to continue. She's probably trying to cooperate with all the parts at the same time. She teaches me that the parts can get together and meet. I practise. It's difficult, but sometimes it works.

In the denying one's world, it's me against them: the doctors, psychologists, public agencies and care system. She doesn't want to go to TT at all. She avoids letting the therapist come close. Deep down, I'm very lonely and far too terrified to bond, to dare trust anyone. Getting close feels awfully dangerous.

When our youngest daughter is four years old, I give birth to my fourth child. I'm very happy with the baby boy, but feel restless. I need to wind down, from top to bottom gear. I have time to reflect, and the insight comes over me with full force: I definitely have various parts inside me.

The parts are in here. They make themselves heard and are a drain on my strength. My thoughts whirl around and their wills pull in different directions. When the parts tear me apart, I feel severely anxious. In the end, I hold a meeting with myself and decide to really give the therapy a proper chance.

The soldier in me

Gradually, I learn more and more about how I can calm the parts down when they're at war. Hurtful memories are released. It's agony, but we deal with them in portions. Reliving events and feelings brings up much pain that has been stored in me. Afterwards, I feel somehow liberated. I feel it's good for me.

When I get help in contemplating my life, I see myself as a prisoner in old patterns. No one protected me when I was small and vulnerable. To survive, my brain created strategies that helped me through fear, pain and humiliation. My various parts had to bear differing experiences because there was no other way out. Inside, I'm a crazy puzzle of bizarre pieces that didn't fit together.

Now the pieces are slowly falling into place. I'm becoming aware of the situations in which the various parts become active, and understand that I'm doing to myself exactly what others have done to me: driving myself very hard, condemning myself and so on. After decades, it feels almost impossible to break the vicious circle. It takes time and effort to understand and change.

I'm dependent on other people's approval. I charge my batteries with praise for my skill at work, in the kitchen and in the club I belong to.

The part of my personality that controls my life in so many ways is the hard-driving one. When she takes over, I become like a soldier, going into a kind of vacuum, determined to go on and on, at any cost. That part of me feels nothing: no fear, no joy and no grief.

That pushy, goal-oriented side is my fuel. Thanks to her, I've survived my hardest years. The driving one managed to rescue my son when he was kidnapped, and enabled me, when our daughters were little, to do everything in my power to save them from having as hard a time as Matteo had done. She helped me in my work, my leisure interests and my quest to find out what had really happened. She has made me feel invulnerable.

Dad's legacy

Nevertheless, it's devastating when the hard-driving part takes over completely. Then she doesn't help me, and makes me feel very bad. Then I work and struggle, exceed my limits and neither eat nor rest. I get facial tics and my whole body trembles. She constantly mixes up what's happening in the present with experiences from the past.

I've often been self-destructive. I've sacrificed myself for my children. Forced myself to polish the whole house until it's shining clean before feeling I've deserved to eat. I switch off my hunger and my needs. The hard-driving part of me has been in charge when I made the wrong choices in life — when I've shut down my feelings, been deaf to the warning bells and returned to my violent former partner, for example. Now I understand how I could agree to be deceived by him again and again. The hard-driving one took over completely and solved everything in her own way.

Unfortunately, the hard-driving one is strengthened by society's prevailing norms. You're supposed to be diligent and efficient. Rush on, struggle and not examine your own feelings. Work hard to be rewarded, to be accepted.

I feel Dad's legacy. His driving side dominates me completely. He feels nothing for his women, children or employees. Nothing. The money and achievements come first, not the people. This legacy is devastating for me and others.

A clear example is when I organise an event at the children's sports club. Enterprisingly, I persuade the volunteering parents to do this and that. I become ice-cold and rock-hard to make things happen. Too late, I discover I'm using the same domination techniques as my father. I become as driving and insensitive as my father used to be as an employer and family father. That's a terrible realisation.

The scared child

The sad part of my personality hasn't been allowed to take up space. She has hardly been able to help me survive all the injustices and violence. If the sad one had been allowed to take over completely, I would never have had the strength to live. And I wasn't allowed to be sad around Dad, either. I had to be grateful and diligent. So the sad part was suppressed and became a lump in my stomach. I can't really allow myself to be sad. Instead, I get shaky and anxious, with a stomach-ache.

When I react strongly to something that's happening now, it's often my inner child, the scared child, who is experiencing fear or danger. That part of me is small and terrified. When she takes over, I lose the ability to be an adult. She lives on in my old terror of adult power, and lacks the ability to make mature decisions.

It's as if the whole of me is kidnapped by my inner child. I'm totally in my own world and feel extremely tense, convinced something terrible will happen to me — that my child will die, for instance. The fear spreads, as cold as ice, throughout my body, from the feet up. Feelings of vulnerability, powerlessness and despair take over completely. It becomes like when I was in the mental hospital. Then, the scared child and the sad part were probably fully switched on all the time.

I don't understand why my feelings are so intense. When my daughter isn't allowed to play an important match, I react as if *I* were the one who had ended up on the substitutes' bench. I react with strong emotions, as if I've been rejected, am suffering and have to defend myself. Then, for a while, I would behave like a defenceless child, instead of the adult mother who should be there for her daughter.

Blackout

Places can awaken the scared child. A visit to the neighbourhood around Dad's restaurant gives me a powerful, sickly feeling of discomfort in my stomach. Scents also trigger the scared part of me. The repellent smell of stale beer at the pub reminds me strongly of nasty situations I've experienced at Dad's restaurant. Once, I get into a fight with a pub bouncer. When he grabs me, I dissociate completely. I have flashbacks and disappear from the reality of here and now, away from my adult self.

The bouncer and the pub turn into my threatening father at the restaurant; I fly back in time to moments when I was a threatened, terrified child. Panic-stricken, I struggle as the bouncer wrestles me to the floor. He's strong. I haven't a chance. I lie there and my whole body shakes. His grip is superhumanly hard, the weight on my chest increases and it feels like all the air is being squeezed out of my lungs. There's buzzing in my ears, I gasp for breath and fight for my life. I don't know what I'm doing. Everything around me turns black. Afterwards I, the adult everyday woman, have a big memory gap. I stand there, totally bewildered, with a massive swollen lip and a report of violence against an employee.

The hard-driver part finds the scared child extremely provocative. As long as the hard-driving part keeps me shielded and fully occupied, the scared child disappears into the dark. There's no room for her.

Fury

Through the therapy, I get to know the angry part of my personality. For a long time, I haven't dared to acknowledge her, and I've forgotten a lot that happened when she took over. That's been far too dangerous to know. When I've felt stressed, I've got worked up and lost my grip on time and space.

I realise that my anger has been frightening for my children. I want them to feel safe. In the therapy, I learn to leave the children for a while when the angry part starts up. That's better, and I'm glad they have a good father.

When the pressure has become extreme, I haven't reacted by getting angry, I've become *super angry!* So inhumanly angry that I haven't been able to control myself. Like an explosion! In the past, I wanted to shoot my father and I wished Nicolas would disappear forever. Then, I stopped in the middle of the motorway and yelled at my husband to get out of the car.

My rage lives in my heart. When the angry part gets going, the palpitations start, my pulse rises and I break into a cold sweat from the adrenaline surge. In therapy, we talk about it being okay to be angry, but not to do anything when you are. I see now that my feelings are very messy. If I get terribly angry like that, I get sad. And I get angry because of the sadness… and sad because of the anger…

Another, more forceful and furious part of my personality doesn't care at all about what others think. When that part takes over, I simply don't give a toss about other people. It's me against the world! I've been treated so badly that I have the right to take back what's mine. All the same, I can be frightened of this part. Under severe duress, I get a blackout and it takes control completely. Afterwards, I don't know what I've done.

Disaster

I'm burdened by a lot of shame and self-critical thoughts. One part of me is as judgemental as Dad. She treats me as badly as my stepmother and Dad have always done. Tormenting me. Pushing me down. Showing disgust and contempt. Making me feel ashamed and guilty. The feeling is in my stomach and head.

The judgemental part tells me everything is my own fault. That I'm not good enough. She wants me to believe I was born to be a slave and should blame myself. She whispers to me that it's my own fault that my uncle abused me sexually. I was pretty, and after all I stayed there and didn't stop him...

The judgemental one creates a great deal of anxiety and robs me of my strength. She paints a mental picture of impending disaster. There'll be chaos at work; everything's my fault and I'm going to get fired. I have nightmares that my children will die and that it's my fault I didn't manage to protect them.

The judgemental part attacks others too. My daughter's puberty triggers me. I'm thrown back to the time to when I was her age, and I realise too late that I sound just like my stepmother, condemning my daughter in the same harsh words I had to hear myself. Now, that hardly ever happens, and if it did, I've learnt to repair it afterwards. There's a big difference now.

Now and then

The work of assembling all the voices requires my full concentration. When one part of my personality takes over, I'm not aware of the others at first. It's very messy inside me. *Okay*, I think, *now let's sit down together at the same table. If all the parts cooperate, everything will go much easier.*

Things are moving forward. I really trust my therapist now, although the judgemental part still wants to trick me into doubt sometimes, when she's unsure and in full swing. Gradually, I see that two of my parts feel like victims: the sad part and the scared child. The others — the angry, judgemental and hard-driving parts, and the one who is fighting the world — seek control.

The various parts of my personality are kind of left behind in the past, when I became traumatised. So they misunderstand the events I'm involved in now, as an adult, and mix them up with experiences in childhood and adolescence. In various ways, they try to protect me from the terrifying old experiences they think are happening *now*. Things can be totally crazy when they are in control.

I'm becoming increasingly aware of how judgemental I am towards myself. I see how I torment myself, just as I'm used to everyone else doing to me. During the therapy, I get help in untying the knots, one at a time.

TT teaches me techniques I can apply when my thoughts trigger dissociation and feelings of panic. I practise getting back to the present by using my senses. At first it's very difficult, but in time I become ever better at discovering what's going on in me. I stop, breathe and listen for everyday sounds that help me to stay present. Turning on the radio and listening to the news becomes a way of feeling that I'm not back in the old traumatic period. *I'm living here and now!*

Distrust

My children are my great joy. Seeing them being happy is my best medicine. My kids are my jewels!

I get involved in their sports club. That's fun. I enjoy myself, and before long I'm put in charge of sports for the whole club. After a year, I'm recruited to a major sports association.

I'm working half-time. At the same time, the therapeutic process is going on intensively. I certainly am enterprising. That's my legacy from Dad. The sure knowledge that I've survived all the trauma has made me strong. I know what I want and find ways to reach my goals. But without the therapy, I would never have managed.

Living with post-traumatic stress and dissociation is hard. It's difficult for both me and my family when I lose touch with reality here and now. I disappear into myself, into feelings from old traumas that kidnap my body and brain.

I've spent many years practising the ability to not feel. I survived by shutting down. Switching myself off. Disappearing. It's a big challenge to practise feeling and dare to remain in strong feelings like anger, fear and sorrow. Overcoming the terror is a long journey.

I've never been in love. Never acted out any lust. I can like someone, but stay cold. I simply don't fall in love. It bothers me that what has happened still affects me so much. I find it hard to trust anyone fully. If my husband praises me, saying, *'What a good job you've done!'*, I become suspicious and spontaneously think: *What's he after now?* That hurts me so much...

Hounded

My strong will puts a strain on my body. All the time, I'm living with an inner frustration, an extra load of stress that impairs my memory and makes it hard to unwind. Why do I forget so much? I look despairingly for the keys and finally find them in an odd place, maybe in the fridge. I don't remember that I've already been shopping for bread and milk, so I go back to the shop and buy the same things again. My brain's in overdrive and I'm ashamed of being so forgetful. In the evening, I lie awake brooding about what to do. The anxiety grinds on. I get palpitations, feel hounded and can neither eat nor sleep.

During the therapy, the penny finally drops: no wonder it's so messy inside my head! I do the vacuuming, think about my job, ponder over the meeting I'm going to attend and answer my children's questions — all while being totally absorbed by chaotic perceptions and feelings from the past. I struggle to exert some control, but become fragmented and confused in the present.

I'm learning to deal ever better with the frustration in stressful situations, and take care of myself. Before, I used to sacrifice myself for my kids. Everything I felt was vicarious, through the children. I was unable to feel anything for myself. Now I'm cracking the code: *if I take care of myself and make sure I feel well, then my kids feel good too. It's okay to feel happiness at times.* Physical exercise, sauna and hot baths help. Now I sleep much better. I'm still forgetful, but mislay perhaps a tenth compared with before: a marked improvement. I stop taking all medication, except the odd sleeping pill sometimes. I manage without them. That's important.

In the old world

Now I can start looking back at my childhood. I can remember the contexts and gradually find a common thread, rather than just fragments. I realise I was just a housemaid. I was there, with my father and stepmother, to be useful. They gave me no love. I didn't get it then, but I see it clearly now and the realisation is painful.

I rarely meet my brother. I love him enormously, but being in touch is too painful. We remind each other of all the hard times. He feels bad and is by no means strong enough to think about what happened.

For our half-siblings, it is different. They were able to live with their own mother, after all, and were well treated. But my little sister is mentally ill. Although she was given everything she fancied when she was little, she hates her mother. She saw how terribly badly our father and her mother treated me. I was there when her mother was stabbed by Dad, and became a little bit like a mother to her. I'm still her saviour. When she feels bad, I'm the one who can take her to the psychiatric emergency clinic. I'm closer to her than anyone else. She knows I too have been down in the darkest depths and has confidence in me.

We don't choose our parents. Unfortunately, I got a very sick father. He has executed two people, severely stabbed another, and beat and exploited many. And he has hurt me very badly. As children, we are totally dependent on our parents. It's impossible to live without them, so we adapt. We get brainwashed.

I want as little as possible to do with old neighbours and others from the past. If I meet someone, I can instantly feel how he or she reacts: *Oh, it's HER, HIS daughter. What a tragedy!* I feel terribly vulnerable and don't want to set foot there, in the old world.

Meeting Grandpa

I decide to travel to France to finally find my mother's family, far up in the mountains. As a mother, I want to search for my roots and those of the kids. As I swing past the last bend in the road, I see the green valley spread out in front of us. My mother's aunt is obliging to me. This old peasant woman is incredibly like me. The same nose, the same hair... that feeling's very special. My unknown origin is here. The link to my mother.

When I meet my grandfather, I understand that he, just like me, has been living with a lie about Mum's death. He didn't know the truth about the murder either. When the death news came from Sweden, he was told that my father had shot my mother dead, but that it was her own fault. Grandpa was told she'd been unfaithful many times. Dad was said to have caught her and her lover in the act and killed them without premeditation.

Over the years, that lie has weighed on my grandfather with dark shame. According to the traditional way of regarding women, he gave away his daughter to my father, and then she brought disgrace on her husband. Grandpa had to live with this 'truth' year in and year out, until he became an old man.

Grandpa is a simple, wise person who radiates calm. When I've told the truth, I arrange for both him and my uncle to come to Sweden, to stay with me and visit the cemetery where Mum's buried. It makes amends, emotionally. Grandpa faints at the grave. All tension is released. Later he says, *'I'm a rich man now. I've got my daughter back.'* A year later, Grandpa dies. It feels good to know that he died in peace. I'm proud of myself that I was able to contribute to that.

Healing wounds

It's still hard to really allow myself to be sad. Then it feels like I've lost. When Grandpa dies, I react physically. My pulse races and I get asthma and shortness of breath. My sadness comes out in that way, by me getting angry and stressed, rather than sorrowful.

One thing I'm working on is learning to live with my hypersensitivity. Accepting it as a scar from old wounds. Maybe I even benefit from it. My antennae are extremely well developed. My trauma has taught me to read other people. I suss them out and know exactly what their intentions are. It's like a sixth sense.

Just like many others who have suffered, I react strongly when people are in distress. When I see beggars outside the grocery store, I get deeply affected. It's like seeing my own grandfather standing there and digging in the rubbish bins for cans to cash in.

I used to apologise for my existence. Now I've started living one step at a time, and can indulge myself in feeling really good, and every so often even experiencing joy. I'm learning to see myself as a valuable person with the same rights as everyone else. And I'm learning to trust the right people — those who really wish me well.

These days I feel strong, but am still very sensitive. Every day, it's a challenge to make everyday life work. I'm focusing on keeping myself in the moment. If I get stressed I easily fall into old patterns, but now I have methods that work. It's vitally important to take time to breathe. Spirituality is my friend. Praying helps me to take a break, focus inwardly and create stillness. That gives me a good feeling.

My new family

I feel best of all when I'm with my uncle in France. I can be my true self there, and find the serenity in my soul. Everything goes in slow motion. When we get there, I sleep for three days. There's no stress there. I think I enjoy it so much because I find what I've missed most of all: family fellowship and a social context where you're valued based on who you *are*, not what you *do*. That's what I've lacked and longed for. It's so much more important than material things, and can't be bought for money.

The most important thing to me is to break destructive patterns so they aren't transferred to the next generation. My uncle's incredibly humble and loving. The children play and get lots of kisses and hugs. Getting the sense of belonging in a real family, despite all the terrible things that have happened, is like winning the jackpot. The scars will always remain in me, but deep healing is under way.

I'm bitter about how society has managed my and my brother's lives: the social welfare authorities, health services, the social insurance office... I've felt raped! Their systems have made me ill.

A meeting at the social insurance office feels like sitting in the dock as a defendant in a trial. I go around with a nasty feeling in my stomach. I feel stressed about not being believed, and about the truth never emerging. I've suffered so much — what a high price I've had to pay!

Those public agencies should never have handed us over to our father. He murdered our mother and abused us mentally and physically. But no one wanted to see the truth.

A mistake is made. For the vulnerable small kid, it has lifelong repercussions. What on earth were they thinking? I just don't get it.

Vindictive

Many people believe all this happened in a different country, but it happened here in Sweden. That's the very hardest thing to take in. I was born a Swedish citizen in Sweden and grew up here. Yet I was totally at the mercy of the system.

Dad shot Mum — in Sweden!

We were returned to Dad — in Sweden!

I was treated like a slave and raised to be a thief — in Sweden!

And I've spun around in the care merry-go-round for many years, without getting the right help — in Sweden!

Deep down, I'm furious because Dad robbed me of my childhood. He deprived me of Mum. He stole my trust. In fact, he took *everything* away from me. I'm furious about him brainwashing me with a completely different 'truth' about our mother and family. Livid because I was accused of making everything up, although it was all true. Outraged that my own father caused so much anguish and pain.

The sorrow can wash over me all of a sudden. With no warning, when I'm sitting in the car and driving somewhere on an everyday errand, I can become terribly sad about everything that's happened and all I've missed out on. Now I'm in touch with my own feelings and feel indescribable sadness. I may still feel vengeful because Dad's a wealthy, free man, pulling new women into his destructive life. But I'm working on creating a distance between us. Dad is living on with the past, but I've moved on.

Forgiving myself

A grim upbringing leaves its scars. For me, the shame and self-accusations have been the worst. I've been incredibly ashamed of decisions that have led to disastrous situations for me and my eldest son. I've been ashamed about how I repeatedly trusted Nicolas, although he'd deceived me so many times.

Today, I've forgiven myself for things I did as a child, such as going back to Dad in Stockholm instead of staying at the family home in Skåne. He was my father, but also Mum's killer. How could I love a murderer? Coming to terms with that is hard.

I grew up in a sick family that I myself hadn't chosen. I did my best and never wanted to ruin things for either myself or my children. What we've never been helped to learn, or understand, we can't create by ourselves unaided. This is an important insight. We shouldn't judge ourselves so harshly.

I haven't fully reconciled myself to everything, but I'm practising it. Trying. Learning. I get terribly sad when I think about what's happened. The feelings catch up with me. I'm mourning my childhood now, but I'm *feeling*. I'm not shut down, and I'm not being tossed about by dissociative parts that seize control of me.

My youngest child is just four years old. When I look into his eyes, I see how vulnerable small kids are — how dependent on the adults taking care of them and showing them what's right and wrong. At that moment, there's a deep sadness inside me. I sit down and play with him, as no one ever did with me in my childhood. I've been aloof in the past, but now I'm learning how to play with my child.

The shame lifts

It hurts when I think about my own childhood. I've faced a lot of pain in life, and suffered a great deal. My father, who should have been my protector, betrayed me. My uncle, who should have protected me too, was another betrayer. I now understand I was especially vulnerable to being let down and exploited. No wonder Nicolas also let me down and treated me badly. Even if he wasn't aware of it, he could easily see I made an excellent victim for his power needs. I was so used to being exploited, and I'd never learnt to make out who I could trust.

It's liberating when the shame lifts. What happened can't be erased. I'll bear the scars for the rest of my life, and I still carry the grief in my stomach, but I see that I've accomplished a lot, out of nothing, and am doing my best for the kids.

I used to feel everything would collapse if I thought about myself. Gradually, I'm learning how to allocate my energy so that it lasts in the long run. I take time out when life spins too fast. I breathe, let go, relax and restart.

I'm managing to integrate my childhood experience more and more with the Felicity I am today. The scared child and the angry, sad, judgemental, hard-driving and vindictive parts are getting closer to one another and beginning to merge. That's making me ever stronger.

Now and again, the various parts of my personality can still be triggered, but it's increasingly rare. A challenging activity gets the hard-driving one started. But now I'm aware of my patterns, see connections and can act differently. No part takes over, and I don't get knocked out. There are no watertight partitions among us. Sometimes we're one and the same.

United

The change in me is noticeable in my everyday micro-actions. I used to force myself to clean the whole house, do the laundry and wash up without either eating or taking a break. The alarm went off in me and I was ruled by that 'must' feeling. Now, when my mouth is dry, I make sure to drink; I eat when I'm hungry; and if I'm tired I lie down and sleep for an hour — all without feeling worthless.

In the past, when I got angry, I used to be carried away by the anger. Everything else disappeared. When I was sad, I was really, really sad, completely immersed in deep sorrow, and ended up in no-man's land. Now I can be sad without the rest of me shutting down. Without falling into the pit of despair.

I sometimes used to have intense outbursts against my son. I would get furious and let it rip. I didn't understand what was happening, or why I was reacting so strongly. Then I felt ashamed, tidied up after myself and asked for forgiveness. Now I can handle my anger better. The children notice I've become more secure. The eldest ones know I'm in therapy and are aware of my sensitivity.

I have a great need to be alone and can even go to a café by myself. It used to be impossible to sit there calmly on my own. The part that made it impossible took over completely. Now I'm united instead of split. I trust myself and can even enjoy sitting there and having a coffee alone, in peace and quiet. Quite simply, I'm pleased with myself. I deserve to take a break and feel good.

Somehow, finally, I'm reconciled to my existence. Now, in mid-life, I think, *Shit, I've tormented myself so much! Hell, what a lot I've been through!* It's sad to grasp how bad things have been but, using my experience, I'm building the future. It's okay to be different, to be sensitive, to be sad sometimes. But I've discovered I stay balanced and feel whole when all the parts inside me virtually melt into one. That's happening more and more often. Several parts that used to exist have completely disappeared. Not long ago, there were just four of us. Now there are three.

Recovery

Despite my great progress, I still feel exhausted. Eventually it turns out that I'm suffering from an illness that makes me extra sensitive to stress. It causes fatigue, anxiety, despondency, insomnia, a short fuse, heart palpitations, tremors, weight loss and other diffuse symptoms that can easily be confused with exhaustion, depression and eating disorders. So the disease can be difficult to detect. Research shows that it may be associated with long-term stress and severe trauma. It affects the whole body — not just the metabolism, but also brain function and both mental and emotional health.

The doctor tells me I need an operation. With all my unpleasant experience of the care services after abuse and mental-health problems, it's an ordeal to be hospitalised again. But I've got so far in my treatment that I manage to surrender myself to the anaesthesia staff and let go of control. I succeed in coping with the pain after the surgery, remaining in hospital and trusting the staff. That's proof that I've come quite a long way in gaining enough courage to trust.

The postoperative period feels like a new chapter in my life. I sleep better, my appetite improves and I feel happier and more alert. The operation simply makes me feel much better and gives me emotional stability. Living feels easier.

Standing up for myself

One day, my eldest son comes home and tells me he's bumped into my father in town. Matteo recognises his grandfather and goes up to him. But my father shows no pleasure in seeing his grandchild. Immediately, he demands Matteo's help, there and then. Matteo doesn't have time and replies that he has to catch a train. Dad gets angry and accuses him, saying: *'You're as lazy as your mother.'*

Matteo's story makes my blood boil. My father — as disrespectful as always! Simmering inside, I lift the handset and dial his number. It's time to put an end to it.

I make it clear to Dad that I haven't forgiven, and will never forgive, him for killing my mother. I tell him I haven't forgotten that he's murdered two people; beaten and manipulated his women and children; and betrayed me cruelly.

Dad is insolent. He threatens me with divine retribution, dangles the prospect of an inheritance, and says I'll regret my attitude. But I make it clear to him that I don't want his dirty cash. *'I just want one thing from you: distance. Your money's just bits of paper to me.'*

It feels incredibly good to confront him. I'm scared, but proud. I realise this step is necessary. Afterwards, I have a superb sense of relief, but also a heavy sorrow. He's a perpetrator, but my father despite everything. My origin. A component of my early life that has influenced me greatly. I can't erase that.

The confrontation has freed my mind. Since that day, I've been able to focus much more on here and now, and the future. At times, of course, I feel infinitely lonely. When I see the kind of support my friend gets from her mother, when I sense the joy and love that exists between her children and their grandmother — that's when I miss my own mother most acutely. It's like a void in my heart. I have a rootlessness and thirst for belonging. The grief and sense of loss are still there, but don't rule my life. That feels very positive.

Guardian angel

I'm entitled to tell my story — to stand up and say who I am and what I've been through. It gives me a sense of redress. Besides, I think it can help others.

I feel that the chance to live with my kids and give them a good childhood is a powerful healing process. It's important to forgive oneself. I want to be honest with the children and answer their questions as best I can. They know their grandfather's a sick man. Kids are clever. They understand he's not a good person to be in touch with.

My life could have gone disastrously. I'm glad to be alive, and realise I've had a guardian angel. Now I'm constantly taking new steps forward. Managing to live in the present moment calls for concentration, patience and practice. I'm learning to enjoy simple things like flavours, scents and rest. I sit at the dining table with my children because it feels good. I enjoy my ability to think, feel and be here, now. My quality of life improves all the time, and a truly healthy life is in sight.

Every day, I thank God that I have four healthy children and we're doing well. The way my life used to be is nothing to be ashamed of. In spite of everything, I've accomplished a lot and I'm proud of myself and my family. This is me!

CHAPTER 14

Ground-breaking research on repercussions of trauma

It is hardly surprising that many people with trauma-related dissociative disorders testify to the fact that, over the years, they have met health professionals who did not understand, or want to understand, their clinical picture. These patients often receive many different and sometimes misleading diagnoses.

DID: more common than we think

Severe dissociative disorder is much more common than one might think. Globally, an estimated 0.5–1.5 per cent of the normal population suffer from dissociative disorders. By way of comparison, only 0.04 per cent are estimated as schizophrenic. In psychiatry, trauma-related dissociative disorder is estimated to account for some 10 per cent of cases, while schizophrenia is estimated to affect only 1 per cent.

At the same time, there is obviously a strong research bias. When we search online for the numbers of research studies carried out on various mental syndromes, the pattern becomes clear. By way of comparison, at the time of writing there have been more than 70,000 studies of schizophrenia but fewer than 300 in the area of DID (source: PubMed.gov).

To name some of the few studies on dissociative disorder to date, there is the research by Haslerud and Knudsen in Norway; in the US, that of van der Kolk, Herman and others; and in the Netherlands, contributions to the field from the likes of Ensink, Boon, van der Hart and Nijenhuis.

Eminent trauma researcher

We had the opportunity to interview the Dutch researcher Ellert Nijenhuis, who wrote the Foreword to this book. He is a clinical psychologist, psychotherapist, world-leading researcher in the field and author or co-author of several books, such as the trilogy *The Trinity of Trauma: Ignorance, Fragility, and Control* and *The Haunted Self: Structural Dissociation and the Treatment of Chronic Traumatization*. The latter has been translated into at least 12 languages. He has been researching trauma-related structural dissociation, for example DID, for many years. Below, we use 'DID' as an umbrella term for all forms of dissociative identity disorder.

Historically, DID has been a controversial diagnosis. The brain studies in which Nijenhuis was a collaborating researcher show that brain scans have revealed how the activity shifts when different dissociative parts of the personality appear. The researchers used PET, EEG and MRI. These activity shifts are thus not something that can easily be fabricated by a patient. The results are ground-breaking since opponents previously argued that patients with a lively imagination invented their own personality parts. This is exactly what the team wanted to study.

In modern research, it is also obvious that PTSD and DID are interconnected, albeit with major differences of degree. Post-traumatic stress disorder and trauma-related structural dissociation are, essentially, phenomena that are strongly reminiscent of each other. In PTSD the ANP (everyday part) and EP (survival part) are dissociated from each other. They are not, however, 'split-off fragments' but, rather, a simple dissociative phenomenon. They encompass one major structure and a much smaller one that have some 'mental contents' that they re-enact. The ANP has a weak phenomenal self-concept, with negative symptoms, strong avoidance and detachment, both bodily and emotional.

According to Nijenhuis, the subject of dissociation is still unpopular at many universities. If the phenomenon cannot be documented sufficiently, it is seen as being notional.

'Quite a few colleagues believe that DID is factitious, and just results from suggestions and role play. We found it important to examine that idea scientifically and, like other researchers, use neuroimaging,' he explains.

Many people are stubborn and stick to their prejudices, Nijenhuis says. But not everyone: there has been an improvement. He and his team work in university settings. But massive worldwide prejudices against DID still exist, he points out.

Research findings: essential reading for doubters

Some of Nijenhuis's research has been done at the University of Zurich's Department of Psychology. Dr Yolanda Schlumpf was the main researcher and the author in the Swiss studies. Professor of Neuropsychology Dr Lutz Jäncke has long been conducting research with brain scanners. Nijenhuis showed him results from his previous research and managed to persuade him to put together a joint study. When the study was completed Dr Jäncke, who had initially been thoroughly sceptical, said he no longer had a shadow of a doubt that the mental disorder DID exists. The research data show the truth.

Nijenhuis as the collaborator of the studies demonstrates that not even professional actors succeed in imitating or simulating DID. Mentally healthy individuals who could fantasise very well, plus actors, were instructed to simulate being an ANP and a fragile EP. They were highly motivated to do so and practised playing these roles. It appeared that these individuals have very different patterns of neural and physiological activation in experimental settings while engaging in particular tasks.

He relates how the researchers instructed actors to simulate two different types of dissociative parts, as in DID. The team also directed women with a high propensity to fantasise — who, according to the critics, should be those who were able to simulate DID — but they were entirely unable to do so. The research team instructed the women how to perform the roles well and asked them to practise acting as the ANP and fragile EP. They were highly dedicated, but it was beyond them: they had very different patterns of brain and physiological activity, although subjectively the actors and highly fantasy-prone women thought they had done well.

The results were published after peer review, which would not have happened if the reviewers had considered them worthless. The reviewers took a very critical look, but the results were so convincing and support the view of DID as a trauma related disorder. The brain-imaging data supported this inference, but provided no evidence for the fantasy model, Nijenhuis says.

The researchers showed that there are distinct differences in the brain activity of different types of dissociative parts of the personality. At brain level, everyday ('Apparently Normal') parts and survival ('Emotional') parts — ANPs and EPs respectively — had different reactions to experimental cues, that relate to and can evoke some of the person's trauma memories.

Nijenhuis and his team used personal trauma scripts. Initial findings from studies in 2003 and 2006 were that ANP and fragile EP had different patterns of neural and physiological activation to these scripts. The results raised questions from other interested parties. Some of them claimed that women with rich fantasy lives could easily imitate the patterns of ANPs and EPs. So the researchers repeated the study with precisely such women, as well as with women who showed little tendency to fantasise. They asked every one of the women to tell them about her most traumatic memory. The women's stories were converted into script that were then recorded as trauma scripts, and they then listened while imitating ANPs and EPs. If it were true that DID is about imagination, suggestibility, roleplaying suggestions and actual roleplay, the researchers reasoned, the most imaginative women should be the ones best able to imitate dissociative parts of the personality. The team's hypothesis was that the women involved would be unable to manage it, and the study published in 2012 showed this. The team even found that another group who were also involved in the study, women with low propensity to engage in fantasy, performed relatively better at simulating features of DID than the high-propensity group. But no one succeeded in imitating the dissociative parts' patterns.

The next phase

In the study, the researchers also hypothesised and found that everyday and survival parts have very similar reactions to neutral memories that they share.

In Zurich, his team —including Dr Yolanda Schlumpf as the main researcher — took the next step: testing a new hypothesis. This was that if ANPs and EPs in DID patients were subjected to stimuli they could not consciously perceive, they would react differently. The team also expected differences between the real DID patients and the control group of simulating actors. This was exactly what happened. The hypothesis was confirmed and the research findings were published.

Nijenhuis devised these studies more than 25 years ago. He was then working in even stronger headwinds as he tried to convey his hypothesis on structural dissociation. Only more recently have the studies been feasible. The facts emerging from this new research may, it is hoped, encourage more people to acknowledge the existence of structural dissociation. The research is now continuing in collaboration with the largest trauma clinic in Switzerland, and the team uses the brain scanner and EEG in Zurich, with Professor Jäncke's help. Nijenhuis is highly impressed by the patients who manage to participate in studies with the scanner.

Only a small group of patients, he told us, can switch between ANPs and EPs (the everyday and survival parts respectively) in a controlled experimental environment, while lying in a brain scanner where their heads are fixed in place. Many of them simply cannot do it because of their past traumas. But those who can and do are extremely brave, and he was very proud of them, Nijenhuis said.

PTSD and DID — deviations on the same scale

Dr Sima Chalavi and her team at the University of Groningen, in the Netherlands, show in their research that brain structure differs between patients with PTSD and DID on the one hand and non-traumatised people on the other. The main differences are in the volume of certain structures. Patients with PTSD and DID exhibit similar brain abnormalities. The team found many differences in brain structures. For example, in both groups, the hippocampus is smaller in size; but the deviation is larger and more distinctive in DID.

Nijenhuis believes that identity is a theme that people often forget when they are discussing PTSD. When patients relive their trauma, they perceive that they are the same people they were when it occurred. They go back to that time and place, and become the victim again. But they also get identity issues of their own at that time. This phenomenology captures the dissociative parts' experiences and conceptions of self, world, and self-as-a-part-of-this-world. 'Who' also concerns an answer to the question of what being a particular dissociative part is like, since only first subjects can answer that question.

'They think the same things about themselves as they did then. They relate to other people as they did then. So from my point of view PTSD and DID are both dissociative disorders, but many authorities in the PTSD area don't seem to like that.

'You could say that the ANP and EP structures are similar but much simpler in PTSD. If they'd been in touch with their present-day selves, they'd feel secure. It would still be an unpleasant memory, but they'd perceive it as the person they are today. But it's not like that. When PTSD patients relive, for example, an accident they had a decade ago, they become the person they were then, and that's an EP.'

Thus, Nijenhuis has presented many conceptual and empirical arguments why PTSD and DID are on the same scale, as a dissociative disorder, but differ greatly in complexity:

(a) ***Normal PTSD*** tends to have an ANP (the predominant everyday structure) and a minor EP (a survival part that is emotional).

(b) ***Complex PTSD*** has a slightly more distinct ANP and more than one EP — not particularly developed, but nonetheless present.

(c) **Minor DID ('OSDD')** usually has an ANP, but also perhaps another, minor ANP that is activated sometimes, and two or more EPs that have become more developed. These are even more distinct and separate parts that increasingly often take over the individual's actions. They can be more isolated from one another.

(d) **Major DID** has more than one clearly separated ANP and several EPs, and many of them can be highly developed, separate parts combined in a wide range of ways, in highly variable numbers and modes of functioning and interacting.

There are of course numerous variations, but this is the basic scale, Nijenhuis believes:

We compared brain activity in PTSD patients and DID patients. I show which areas are involved when the patients start functioning at EP level, and which are active when they're at ANP level. The studies reveal huge similarities across the board, for traumatisation of all the various degrees of severity, PTSD and DID — similarities that can't be random.'

More than our brain cells

Today, the brain and neurosciences are hot topics. Neuropsychology can show us what the brain does, and Nijenhuis believes we have idealised the brain too much:

'Imagine having an image of a person's brain activity and asking a neurologist what the person in the picture was feeling right then. What can the scientist say? Nothing — without knowing what the person was doing and what the surroundings were like.

Believing that the brain alone can explain anything is far too simplistic. That would mean that consciousness doesn't matter.'

Nijenhuis refers to researchers such as Francisco Varela, the Chilean follower in the footsteps of the philosopher Schopenhauer, who asked, *'What would the brain be if there were no conscious people who knew it existed?'* To study the brain and be able to interpret the results, we need consciousness and interest in ourselves in the first place. Moreover, we encompass a body as much as a brain, and are at all times connected with an environment. We are inherently embodied, world-embedded, and social beings.

'We who research the brain need patients' consciousness — that is, their subjectivity. We must listen to them while studying their brains, ask "How do you feel right now?" and then compare the answers with the patterns we see. To make progress in our studies of dissociative disorders, we brain researchers need to collaborate closely with people who know the patients very well, and the patients themselves. All three of these should plan and interpret the studies together. That is a neurophenomenological approach to dissociative disorders. Just looking at images of brain activity and interpreting them without knowing what the person was doing, thinking, feeling and desiring during the brain measurements misses out on the importance of subjectivity.'

Clinicians (i.e. the patients' psychotherapists) can also fulfil an important role in this research.

'Clinicians may need to help patients to clarify and formulate what they experience. That's the role of therapists in a project I would like to set up,' Nijenhuis states.

In 2017, for the research study *Is it Trauma- or Fantasy-based? Comparing dissociative identity disorder, post-traumatic stress disorder, simulators, and controls*, he received the prestigious Pierre Janet Writing Award from the International Society for the Study of Trauma and Dissociation. The year before, Nijenhuis had received the same Award for the first two volumes of his book trilogy *The Trinity of Trauma*.

Brain activity and reaction time

Nijenhuis's research thus shows distinct differences in brain activity between dissociative patients and control groups, and also clear similarities between PTSD and DID. In the Swiss study, unconscious reactions to subliminally presented stimuli, for example in the form of a fleeting image, were studied and the subjects' reaction times were measured. The fact that a stimulus is presented subliminally means that the exposure time is so short that you have no chance to consciously perceive what you see. Abnormal reaction times were found for EPs, but not for ANPs. EPs activated different brain areas including the parahippocampal gyrus, brainstem, face-sensitive regions and motor-related areas.

'Our participants had to look at a computer screen that was totally blank, except for a small blue dot in the middle. The next thing they were able to perceive consciously was that the dot changed colour to yellow. We asked them to press a button as soon as they saw the dot changing colour. What they'd also seen, without being aware of it because we only showed it for 17 milliseconds, was a face. We showed one nonsense image with the features all mixed up, one neutral face and one angry one.'

Nijenhuis says that in his research he usually gets his hypotheses confirmed when he tests them, but this time he was mistaken. Facial expressions are extremely important cues in interpersonal communication. Nijenhuis had thought the angry face would elicit the strongest neural reactions. Instead, the neutral face accounted for the biggest deviation in brain activity.

Neutral face frightening

People with dissociative disorders symptoms are intimately related to a context of unstable and disrupted interpersonal relationships, and there are two ways to interpret the result. According to the first, the neutral face might be experienced as ambiguous. The patient might think, *What is the face showing?* The patients' ANPs had the same reaction time as the control group. Only their EPs were slower, to a statistically significant extent. As a dissociative part of the personality fixed in the traumatic past, fragile EPs may regard neutral faces as untrustworthy and threatening, and thus become hypervigilant when confronted with them, and prepare defensive motor reactions.

The second possible interpretation may communicate affective unavailability of other individuals, such as primary caretakers, to a traumatised child. The DID patients who participated in the study all reported emotional neglect and abuse by family members. Parents' affective unavailability and disorganised attachment in childhood are major predictors of dissociative symptoms in adulthood.

As Nijenhuis points out, there is little need for DID patients to attend to an angry face for long. Things are clear once a face has turned angry.

Important feelings

Modern psychology is extremely focused on cognition. The main concern is thinking. We seem to have forgotten what the philosophers Schopenhauer and Spinoza once taught us: that human beings are, most of all, creatures of affect and feelings. We are made up of desires — we want security, food, communication, appreciation and strength. We are a bundle of wants. Modern psychology must not forget this. Still, in recent times, scientists have started to appreciate the tremendous importance of feelings more.

'We must integrate longing (need and desire), affect, cognition and behaviour, rather than splitting them up. What people think is strongly linked to what they long and strive for. For example, with respect to dissociative disorders, ANPs and EPs think differently because they long and strive to achieve different things,' Nijenhuis concludes.

From science to therapy

He believes that the clinical and empirical evidence for DID is now so strong that those in psychiatric care and research who have opposed the concept must acknowledge the disorder:

'My hope is that a growing number of researchers will take the research findings from complex dissociative disorders seriously. Child abuse and neglect in various forms also gets more attention nowadays. As late as 1976, it was stated in a psychology textbook that incest was a "one-in-a-million" occurrence. We now know that between five and ten per cent of all women are subjected to it. More and more affected men are also stepping forward. With the expanding number of clinics that are beginning to work with trauma patients, the need to learn, and interest in learning, about trauma and its consequences are increasing.'

Interestingly, the basic model of trauma treatment is very similar to the one advocated by psychologist Pierre Janet (1859–1947) several generations ago. Nijenhuis believes that there is stability over time in what does and does not work in therapy for complex dissociative disorders. The basic idea is that the different dissociative parts of the patient's personality should learn to know and appreciate one another better, and cooperate better with one another. However, different dissociative parts commonly have conflicting needs and desires:

For individuals with DID, the conflict of wants can be described like this: "I've got to live in this family and have a day-to-day life. I must relate to these people. And when they abuse or neglect me, I've got to defend myself." As ANPs, they are concerned with daily life and must thus relate to perpetrators as if they were not perpetrators. At the same time, struggling to survive the horrors these people inflict, EPs are in ongoing defence.

'ANPs manage to concentrate on everyday life and escape EPs by avoiding them, but this avoidance can become frail. EPs may start intruding on ANPs with flashbacks, nightmares and strong feelings. These intrusions constitute part of ANPs' symptoms. EPs may start to haunt ANPs just as ANPs have always, more or less, plagued EPs by displacing and isolating them. EPs, so to speak, throw their traumatic and related experiences and ideas into ANPs' domain. Part of the treatment is that ANPs learn to integrate these contents and the EPs. In collaboration with each other, they must learn to accept and realize what happened to them, and rather than recurrently relive the traumatic memories, they must learn to put them in words, so that the painful past becomes a story told, a narrative.'

Memories fall into place

Janet taught us the importance of integrating dissociative parts. They must begin to recognise one another and share knowledge, feelings, physical sensations and behaviours. Traumatic memories must be integrated into the person as a whole.

When all goes well, the patient can finally say:

When I was a child, I suffered abuse and neglect, and it was terrible. I couldn't cope with being present in all the vile experiences at the same time. So I had to divide my personality. That was how I survived. Now I'm an adult. I'm choosing to be with secure people, and they're helping me deal with everything instead. And now I've finally put these memories into the framework that makes up my life, and I feel good.

CHAPTER 15

Last but not least: the costs of treatment

There are very high costs of trauma to society — not to mention the enormous suffering of the individuals concerned. People with only simple PTSD are often on sick leave repeatedly, over and over again, and unable to return to a functioning everyday life. For severely traumatised dissociative people, life is chaotic. Sheer survival is what they are trying to achieve. When we meet them in therapy, they bring numerous different symptoms and many years of pain. The trauma sticks in their chest like hard concrete. Their suffering cannot be measured in money. Their relatives also pay a high price in the form of their own suffering.

Patients in this category often lack the right diagnosis. Their treatment is focused on other diagnoses, such as depression, bipolar disorder or schizophrenia. The patients thus miss out on the specialised trauma and dissociation treatment they need. Our wish is that no doctor, psychotherapist, psychologist or other health professional should prolong these patients' suffering by failing to see and understand their condition and, accordingly, put adequate treatment in place as soon as possible.

Fulfilment of this wish would bring economic advantages for society. Those who bear primary responsibility for healthcare costs should have a strong interest in looking more closely at the potential cost of a person not being diagnosed correctly and receiving appropriate treatment for trauma-related dissociation, compared with one who receives the right help at an early stage.

In a couple of Sweden's neighbouring countries, researchers have estimated the financial implications of providing more staff-intensive, costly care for people with first-episode psychosis. The studies show savings per patient of around EUR 93,000 over time. These estimates were made in major research projects. Corresponding estimates for severely traumatised patients have not, to our knowledge, been carried out either in Sweden or in its Nordic neighbours.

Costs and benefits

Health-economic analysis applies economic theory to health sciences. Finding out what costs and benefits various interventions lead to gives us valuable information that can contribute to more cost-effective use of limited resources. The question is, quite simply, where society's resources provide most benefit.

We asked the health economist Fredrik Gustavsson to make health-economic calculations for three typical cases. He uses calculations like this to evaluate healthcare and other inputs.

The cases in Gustavsson's calculations are fictitious, but similar to those of many severely traumatised patients we encounter in the treatment room. The first two cases concern people who have not received adequate treatment for their complex traumatisation. Unfortunately, there are many such examples in the care sector. The person in the third case was identified in early adulthood, when adequate treatment was put in place.

Correct treatment saves suffering and money

Prolonged brain stress and traumatisation can, as we have shown in previous chapters, leave deep wounds that do not heal of their own accord. With the right treatment, however, people possess a remarkable ability to heal and get well. As the stories in this book show us, dissociative people can recover from even extremely severe traumatisation and dissociation.

In conclusion, Gustavsson's health-economic analysis reveals major differences in costs of care measures. It also shows that the pure social costs are much heavier for patients who receive the wrong diagnosis and treatment.

Case 1: Lottie — 11 years on the healthcare merry-go-round

Lottie was a 36-year-old woman who had received many different diagnoses and treatments over the years. Health professionals failed to understand her problems. She was diagnosed with emotionally unstable personality disorder, depression, generalised anxiety disorder, panic disorder, histrionic personality disorder and more. As a child, she was treated in the Child and Adolescent Psychiatry services a few times, but never dared to tell them what she was going through at home.

Lottie studied at university and worked for six months. Then she fell ill and was on sick leave for 11 years. She sought help at the emergency department of a mental hospital, where suicide-risk assessments were carried out. Sometimes they kept her at the hospital and sometimes she was sent home. On five occasions, she was admitted to a psychiatric clinic.

Throughout her 11 years' sick leave, Lottie was treated in outpatient psychiatric care. She had sessions with a psychotherapist, and sometimes a psychologist, in the psychiatric care services. She received cognitive behavioural therapy (CBT) for panic disorder and depression. Lottie also underwent dialectical behavioural therapy (DBT) treatment when previous treatment had not worked.

Case 2: Mary — pain, eating disorders, suicide attempts

Mary was 33 years old. When she was younger, she spent a few years in casual jobs, did some studying and became an assistant nurse. Her plan was to continue in healthcare. She had very good grades in school and was admitted to medical school, but did not dare to begin. Mary studied a few single-subject courses at university, which came easily for her, but her depression and eating disorder worsened and she was sick-listed for six years. She then received sickness benefit, and had been on that for the past six years.

This woman, too, received many diagnoses: depression, generalised anxiety disorder, bulimia, bipolar disorder and schizotypal personality disorder. At no time was her basic trauma problem identified. Conditions such as autism were investigated in a neuropsychiatric examination, without any such diagnosis. She has fibromyalgia. Mary has attempted suicide twice, both times with pills. Once she was found by a friend, and the other time by a relative. She was rushed to hospital, stomach-pumped and received inpatient care for a couple of days after the suicide attempt.

When she was 23 years old, Mary was treated for her bulimia at a specialist clinic for eating disorders. At first, she was an inpatient for five solid months, in a ward for patients with such severe eating disorders that treatment in outpatient care or day care is deemed insufficient. Subsequently, she attended a 16-week course of group therapy at a day-care unit. Later in life, Mary spent three years in traditional psychodynamic psychotherapy as a psychiatric outpatient. She has also tried many other treatments.

Case 3: Louise — the right help early on

This 23-year-old woman spent part of her childhood being cared for in Child and Adolescent Psychiatry. As a young adult, Louise had already been correctly diagnosed and given both medical treatment and psychotherapy with relatively little delay. For five years, she has received adequate phase-oriented psychotherapeutic treatment, with 40 visits a year to the therapist.

These measures have brought about Louise's gradual recovery. Following an initial period of full-time sick leave, she was on half-time sick leave during the treatment period, and in the final phase her sick leave was reduced to 25 per cent.

Financial comparison: major differences

Health-economic calculations show remarkably large differences among these three typical cases involving women we have called 'Lottie', 'Mary' and 'Louise'. The disparities apply to both healthcare and social costs.

Total costs of care measures were EUR 393,000 for Lottie, EUR 251,000 for Mary and EUR 29,000 for Louise. Costs to society amounted to EUR 627,000 for Lottie, EUR 407,000 for Mary and EUR 107,000 for Louise.

For Cases 1 and 2, treatment at psychiatric clinics accounted for the heaviest care costs by far. For Case 3, psychotherapy was the highest care cost.

Diagnosis, treatment and costs

Both healthcare and social costs were thus considerably higher for Cases 1 and 2 than for Case 3. The decisive difference in Case 3 was that, early in life, Louise received the right diagnosis and treatment. She thus avoided spinning round from one care unit to the next, year after year, without getting the care she needed, while suffering ever more painful effects of her traumatisation and dissociation.

Gustavsson comments: *'From a health-economic perspective, the cost differences among the various cases in this report are an interesting clarification... An important factor in this context was that a correct diagnosis helped to ensure that adequate measures could be initiated at an early stage of the illness, which reduced the number of diagnoses and variety of treatment methods. This resulted in both the care costs and costs to society being considerably lower for the third case than for the other two. The* calculations thus show that there are great financial gains from identifying this category of patients efficiently, first so that appropriate treatment methods can be applied to these patients' sets of problems and, second, to reduce resource use in healthcare.'

Quality of life

Appreciable sums can be saved if people suffering from trauma and dissociation promptly receive the right diagnosis and treatment. Over and above the financial benefits, other values are vital to consider as well. One of these aspects is patients' quality of life. If a correct diagnosis, followed up by adequate care measures, can enhance the patient's well-being and functional capacity for the duration of the illness or contribute to a faster recovery, this in itself is of great value.

Greater well-being for patients has major effects for their loved ones too. People close to them feel better and their quality of life improves. If patients' friends and family can help with domestic tasks or give support in other ways, this also leads to a financial gain in terms of the patients' greater well-being during their periods of illness. However, these aspects have not been included in the calculations in Gustavsson's report, since they are complicated to measure and value, and require more resources than were available for his health-economic analysis.

Everyone gains from the right treatment

The conclusion is that more effective diagnosis and treatment for patients with complex traumatisation provide both financial savings and reduced suffering.

Gustavsson writes: *'Taking into account improved quality of life for these patients and those who are close to them, the benefits may be far greater than those illustrated by the results in this report. All in all, these financial and human benefits thus support development of healthcare planning for this patient category.'*

Hope bounces back

People who suffer often just become numbers in the statistics. This may seem belittling and offensive. Nevertheless, we have chosen to highlight the health-economic aspects in this book. Hearing victims' stories gives a deeper understanding of what traumatisation, dissociation and shortcomings in healthcare mean. Keeping tabs on these costs does not mean calling into question victims' rights to treatment and respect — on the contrary.

We are pleased to note that there is no contradiction whatsoever between patients' need for treatment and society's need to keep costs down. Our interests overlap: the individual, loved ones, employers, care services and, ultimately, taxpayers all benefit from knowledge being disseminated so that we can make the right diagnosis at an early stage and immediately start the right treatment. After all, when we spare people from suffering, we save money too.

Never mind eternity
But give me a place
Here in reality
Another life
In another time
No peace of mind now
...
Give me a place on Earth
No need to be in the sun
Just my own window on the street
That I can open and close
as I please

That is all I need
The only thing
my heart demands
That I find some place
where I can choose between
Peace and quiet

Eva Dahlgren

'There was so much anger in my body. The terror and rage were in every part of me. I used to think I was the only one it had happened to: the assaults, the anxiety, having several parts in me, the confusion. I felt like the loneliest person in the world and lived with my secrets. Now I understand that other people too suffer in these ways. When I think about there being many of us, that it's not just me, the shame releases its grip.

I'm not ashamed of what happened. It wasn't my fault. Responsibility lies with the adults who abused me. In therapy, I found the little child in me and took care of her lovingly. I'll never forget the vileness, but it can no longer hurt me. No spectres from the past are restricting my life, and there is no deep fissure in my soul. Every feeling has space inside me. I'm whole, a whole person. Loved and free.'

Yasmine

LAST WORDS

The book you have now read is about the indomitable human ability to overcome even the most severe traumatisation and finally live our lives free from trauma and dissociation. We cannot be unaffected by what we have been through: no one is. But we need no longer be slaves, oppressed by the ordeals we have undergone in the past. We can overcome our painful history and emerge as victors, as our normal life begins.

Live Now is a sign of the times. The book could never have become reality without six brave protagonists: Emma, Christine, Oscar, Yasmine, Joanna and Felicity. Today, they are all living ordinary, rewarding lives. They were traumatised when they sought treatment. For some, life was an inferno, full of pain, chaos and terror. All six have toiled hard to become healthy. Repeatedly and admirably, they have exerted themselves to move forward and come gradually closer to healing. They have actively changed their life story. In old age, they will be able to talk about the years before their healing, but also about many years since the treatment, when they freed themselves from their previous experience. This new period is a completely different part of their story, in which they triumph over the trauma and have lives filled with active careers, new workplaces, new relationships, marriage, parenthood and, not least, self-respect.

Together, we want to spread awareness of trauma and dissociation so as to improve all traumatised people's chances of receiving the right treatment. The more the healthcare services and other institutions make it routine to ask both children and adults whether they are being, or have been, subjected to violence or abuse, or experienced other difficult events that affect them in their daily life, the easier it will be for everyone who meets people in their work to make responsive listening a habit. Perhaps we can help more traumatised people if we often ask the questions. Perhaps this can be the person's key chance of a good life.

'I understand that having several parts inside you may sound odd and made up. But for me, getting to know my parts has had tremendous healing power. Three parts have become one. Now I'm me, Emma. That's a wonderful, lovely feeling. Split up, I was feeble. United, I'm strong. Memories of the experiences that held me back remain, but they no longer rule me. Life's good. I'm whole. I'm free.'

Emma

'Now I realise all the painful times are over. We can look out through the same eyes, breathe at the same time and smile at the same things. We know we're safe. Before, not all parts knew that. They were isolated on their islands. Now I walk around as one whole person on a steady continent.

'I'm very grateful that I finally got the right help. Now I'm working and taking my place in society. Soon I'll give birth to my child. Gently, the good things in life are filling me up. There are really no words to describe what it's like to be free from my past. I'm alive and well, like an ordinary person.'

Joanna

'I want to tell my story to show what a thoroughgoing change has taken place. Today, what's happening around me no longer feels so important. I can face setbacks and challenges. I don't react nearly as strongly with anxiety and fear. So life is getting easier to live.

'My parts are merging more and more. Before, we weren't even aware of one another. Our mutual discovery terrified us. Now we join in the same situations. Sometimes it feels like we're talking at the same time, with a joint voice, and all three of us feel the same thing. Together, we take a deep breath and enjoy ourselves. Being integrated like this is a really great feeling.'

Oscar

Traumatisation and dissociation are normal human reactions to abnormal events — events of the kind that should never happen to anyone at all. There is absolutely nothing spectacular about our human ability to dissociate. When professionals meet survivors, we must sort out and see *how* severely traumatised the person is. Is complex traumatisation hidden here? Many professionals are currently doing superb work with and for traumatised people, but our wish is for far more of them to want to be good partners to trauma victims, working with them during their necessary, arduous journey forward to a functioning, happy life. The traumatised themselves have a very great deal to teach us. We who are around them need to listen to the knowledge and experience they possess.

We thank you for devoting time and effort to reading our book. Readers wishing to know more are best advised to explore further through in-depth literature on the subject. Reading tips (books and links) may be found at the end of this book.

Knowledge of trauma-related dissociation is growing.

There are an increasing number of studies that support the theory that the effects of trauma can reverberate down the generations through epigenetics.

This science is young, which means it is still generating debate. The discussions remind us a lot of the debate we had around trauma and its consequences during the 1990s. Constant interaction inside us as biopsychosocial beings determines which of our gene expressions can influence our behaviour. As we grow up, our brains are modified by the environment we live in. It has also become clear that our human genes and brain are far more modifiable than we previously thought. Research is an important part of the quest for better care for traumatised people. We truly hope that there will be many more studies on this subject. New advances in knowledge lead to progress that benefits all survivors.

The health-economic calculations you have read about in this book show that there is no contradiction between trauma victims' need for effective treatment and society's desire to keep costs down. We want people who live with traumatisation and dissociation to be given more space and the right resources, in society, care services and their day-to-day lives alike. Then, and with a major expansion of care facilities and specialist clinics, we can get a society that always cares about people with lasting wounds from trauma.

Every winter, we in the Nordic countries ensure that everyone injured on a ski slope promptly receives the care that healing requires. In that situation, we are aware of the nature of reality and we plan health resources based on the expected number of fractures. Similarly, we need to ensure that child and adult traumatisation victims receive the right care, without delay. We need to be well aware of genuine existing needs and provide the necessary treatment. Obviously, we would also like to see investments in preventive work.

Compassion is fundamental to healing. This applies to the people you have met in this book and to everyone who is traumatised, but also to all the other unnamed, but unforgotten sufferers from mental illness. True compassion and self-compassion are fundamental for our well-being in general and mental health, in particular: in this respect, we are all united.

WHOLEHEARTED THANKS

We wish to give warm thanks to everyone around us who made the creation of this book possible.

First and foremost, we want to thank Emma, Christine, Oscar, Yasmine, Joanna and Felicity who so generously shared their life and recovery stories with us, simultaneously teaching us all so much. Without you, there would have been no book. Thanks are due, too, to those who allowed us to quote them elsewhere in the book.

We would like to give special thanks to the health economist Fredrik Gustavsson for his calculations, and to Dr Ellert Nijenhuis, who kindly shared his ground-breaking research and wrote the book's Foreword.

Annica wants to warmly thank all her teachers and patients, who have made her professional development and work possible.

We also wish to express our immense gratitude to everyone who helped by reading the manuscript, reviewing it and contributing to improvements and changes. Among you are professionals, trauma survivors and people who have no personal experience of trauma. We have promised to not name some of you but, though nameless, you are not forgotten. Without your critical reviews and wise opinions, the text would certainly differ greatly from its present version.

Many thanks to those of you who have written comments expressing your reactions to the book.

Last but not least, we would like to thank our families, who lovingly and patiently supported us and allowed us to devote much time and attention to the creation of this book. You have our infinite gratitude.

Christina Lejonöga and Annica Lilja Ljung
Stockholm and Malmö, October 2019

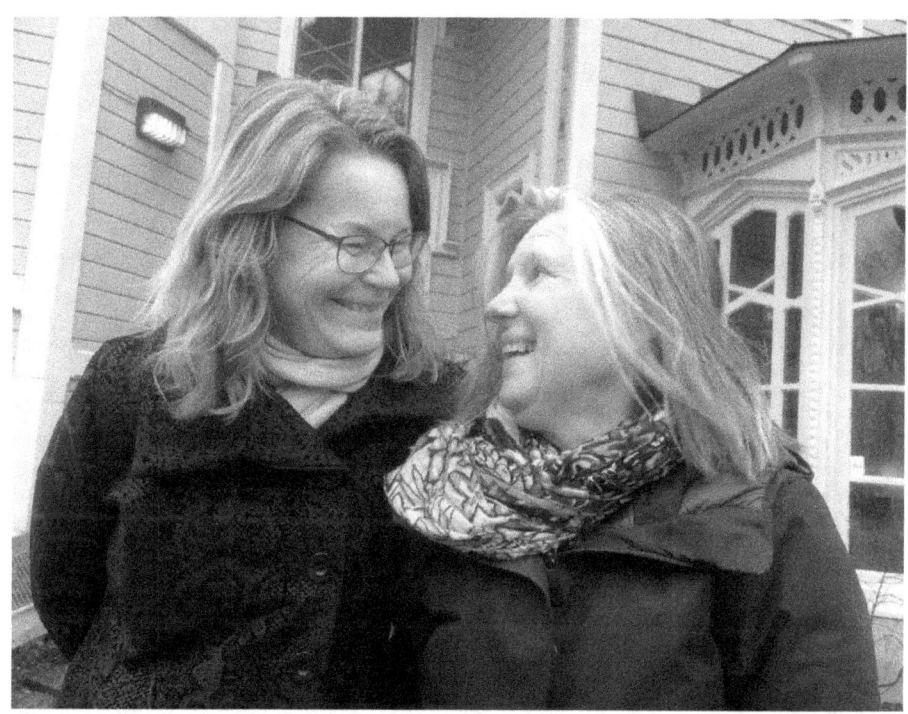

Christina Lejonöga and Annica Lilja Ljung
By Arne Ljung

GLOSSARY

ACT

Acceptance and commitment therapy, a therapeutic method with a set of exercises to assist in various areas of life, such as relationships and work. Patients are helped to stop brooding, and practise their ability to avoid getting stuck in vicious circles of self-accusations, despondency or anxiety. They learn to discover their negative thought patterns and behaviours, accept them and create a sound, functioning sense of commitment beyond the force fields of negative habits.

Action systems

Various biological and emotional systems that dominate every individual's actions on different occasions. The attachment and the threat system are examples of basic action systems. Such action systems are created through interaction among biological, psychological and social factors, such as age, genes, personality and family relationships.

Affect, emotion and feeling

Three words that are often used synonymously nowadays. But they can be, and have been, used in slightly different ways. We have chosen to make both 'affect' and 'emotion' stand for somewhat more fundamental emotional reactions, dominated by biological factors and often powerful. Naturally, they are also influenced by cultural factors and personal experiences, above all in relationships. However, those experiencing the affect or emotion are seldom aware of it. We have used the word 'feeling' for what is often (at least partially) a conscious, subjective experience.

Affect-focused psychotherapy

This includes various methods based on the knowledge that we are all born with a rich set of primary affects (see above). We all have access to these affects, but they are largely unconscious: very often, they govern our thoughts and actions without our being aware of it. In affect-focused psychotherapy, this innate foundation is explored to boost patients' ability to reflect, and learn to use their feelings in a way that is in line with their intentions and wishes. The goal is that they should not be ruled impulsively by their feelings.

Altruistic joy

Disinterested or unselfish pleasure. Without any personal benefit, we can rejoice in the joy and success of others.

Amygdala

Part of the brain that manages strong feelings and stores feelings in the memory. The Latin word *amygdala* means 'almonds'. The amygdala is composed of two small almond-shaped regions in the limbic system that help us identify threats and warn of danger. They play an important role in our ability to feel fear, terror, etc., and are highly involved in stress. The amygdala adjusts, for example, breathing, blood pressure and heart activity.

ANP

Abbreviation for 'apparently normal personality' — the 'ordinary' and seemingly well-functioning dissociative part. One and the same person can develop several ANPs. For the sake of simplicity, we have chosen to call ANPs 'everyday parts'.

Attachment patterns

These are shaped in infancy. From birth, we learn to relate to the people in immediate proximity to us. Patterns are created that we unconsciously continue to follow in our close relationships for the rest of our lives. Through research, these attachment patterns have been divided into groups, to enable us to understand and work on them. Encouragingly, these patterns can be modified. People who have not developed a secure attachment pattern can acquire it through psychotherapy. Creating this attachment enables them to live in well-functioning relationships.

Behavioural system

From birth, infants are governed by instinctive behaviours aimed at getting their basic needs met. Attachment is one such innate behavioural system, its purpose being to give the child security and closeness.

Behaviourism

An early school of psychology based on the idea that human behaviour can be studied objectively, without reference to inner mental experience, and focusing on how our behaviours are affected by the environment. Stimulus and response are key concepts. Behaviourism does not take into account our free will, memories, thoughts or feelings since these, not being directly observable, are not considered sufficiently scientific. Neither the workings of our mind and consciousness nor complex behaviours can be described with behavioural terminology.

Biopsychosocial

The biopsychosocial model represents a holistic view that our health reflects the interplay among biological, psychological and social factors. Biological factors include age and genes. Psychological factors are a matter of identity, personality, etc. Examples of social factors are close relationships and group affiliation.

Bipolar disorder

A psychiatric diagnosis in the DSM system, also known as manic depression, characterised by marked mood swings between depression and mania. Between episodes the person has healthy periods, often lasting several years.

Borderline personality disorder

A psychiatric diagnosis in the DSM system, characterised by rapid mood swings from tranquillity and joy to anxiety or despondency. The disorder creates difficulties in close relationships.

CBT

Cognitive behavioural therapy is psychotherapy aimed at identifying and stopping old patterns of behaviour, with patients being trained in using new action patterns to alleviate their mental problems. Cognitive behavioural therapy, cognitive therapy and psychodynamic therapy are all methods derived from theories about human beings and our development. Today, these methods have learnt from one another but remain theoretically and historically distinct.

Cerebral cortex

The outer layer of the brain, consisting of a folded surface 3–5 mm thick, containing billions of neurons. Here, impulses are transmitted back and forth, making us react, think and act.

Cognition

The human ability to learn, think, decide, solve problems, remember, plan and process information, and other rational processes in the human brain.

Compassion

The capacity for sympathy and empathy — emotional and cognitive — with other people, and the desire to actively help relieve their suffering. Our compassion can be trained.

Complex PTSD

Complex post-traumatic stress disorder; see OSDD.

Contemplative neuroscience

A growing field of research where meditation is combined with neuroscience to obtain greater knowledge of our mental abilities. The significance of meditation for compassion, mindfulness, body awareness and our ability to change are studied. These studies have provided important insights that the brain is far more plastic than was previously thought. This means that we humans can develop and change considerably more than we used to think possible.

DBT

Dialectical behaviour therapy, a method of treating emotionally unstable personality disorder.

DDNOS

Dissociative disorder not otherwise specified, a disorder in the structural dissociation category. A person diagnosed with DDNOS suffers from even more severe traumatisation than in complex PTSD and needs professional treatment to attain a healthy life. As for complex PTSD, a correct diagnosis is important, since treatment that is too assiduous in exposing a person's traumatic past can cause retraumatisation. The diagnosis is included in the DSM system and is also called 'Minor DID'.

DESNOS

See OSDD.

DID

Dissociative identity disorder, the most severe traumatisation type, is a serious psychiatric condition involving structural dissociation. Patients present with many symptoms and have several dissociative parts of the personality, arising from different periods of their lives. People are often unaware of their multiple identities. Incorrect treatment can have serious consequences and cause retraumatisation.

The DID diagnosis, which is included in the DSM system, is also known as Major DID. Up to 1994, the condition was called multiple personality disorder. One important change is that DID is no longer categorised as a personality disorder; rather, it now counts as a stress-related mental disorder.

Dissociation

Umbrella term for several symptoms that can manifest themselves in various ways. The symptoms often follow traumatisation and may mean that people suddenly appear absent or 'disconnected', and do not hear or see what is happening in their immediate environment. In its most severe form, 'structural dissociation', fragmentation of the person results, with splitting into two or more coexisting parts over time. If there is dissociation, it is vital to ascertain its scale so that a correct diagnosis is made, since treatment that is too assiduous in exposing a person's traumatic past can cause retraumatisation.

Dissociative identity disorder

See DID.

Dissociative part

To survive, traumatised people can develop more or less isolated parts of their personality, like small islands in a large sea. Every dissociative part of the personality has its own understanding of the world's reality and sense of identity. Clearly separated parts have completely different ways of functioning and can take command of the person's perceptions and feelings. See also Subsystem, ANP and EP.

Dissociative symptoms

Dissociation can manifest itself in single symptoms, such as memory gaps, or in numerous ones. If there are many, the dissociation is more pervasive in the person and is termed a 'disorder'. Dissociative symptoms can be triggered by sensory impressions and thoughts that remind the person of previous traumatic experiences.

DSM system

The Diagnostic and Statistical Manual of Mental Disorders — a diagnostic classification system that originated in the US and is used in psychiatry in several countries. ICD (the *International Classification of Diseases and Related Health Problems*) is the World Health Organization's (WHO) equivalent to DSM.

Dualistic

A dualistic approach is one that rests on two opposing fundamental principles. The expression comes from philosophy, where dualism means a division of reality into two realities of fundamentally different kinds that require different explanatory models, such as body and soul.

Dynamic therapy

Umbrella term for theories and methods in psychotherapeutic treatment, individually tailored to those who seek treatment. Psychotherapists help patients to explore their life situation, relationships, needs and feelings, and to understand their motives and connections with their life stories. The purpose is to increase the patients' awareness, thereby improving their scope for influencing their own lives to a greater extent.

ECT

Electroconvulsive therapy, also called electrical treatment. A treatment type used for several mental illnesses, most often severe depression.

EEG

Electroencephalography, a way to record certain patterns of brain activity. Nerve cells use electricity to transmit information. One way that scientists study EEG recordings is by looking at different waves in the EEG to research different phases during sleep, meditation etc.

Ego states

A healthy, integrated person can struggle with several conflicting desires that are not well integrated. These ego states are not at all the same as the phenomenon of dissociative parts. A person with dissociative personality disorder is divided into many more sharply defined parts, all of whom have their own sense of who they are, the ways of the world and how they relate to their surroundings.

EMDR

Eye movement desensitisation and reprocessing, a type of therapy for trauma treatment developed by Francine Shapiro (US). EMDR is a powerful method that works well in simple PTSD and PTSD. In cases of more severe traumatisation, EMDR can be used as part of a more extensive treatment, provided that the psychotherapist has the right education and experience.

Emotion

See Affect.

EP

Emotional personality — one or more emotional parts that retain strong feelings linked to their painful memories. These dissociative parts try, in various ways, to escape the memory of what happened. For the sake of simplicity, we have chosen to call EPs 'survival parts'.

Epigenetics

A field of genetic science that explores changes in gene expression due to environmental influences. Our human genome contains some 25,000 genes that can either be switched on (expressed) or off (not expressed) during our lives. Many genes can also be more or less expressed in various cells. There is an 'epigenetic memory' that is heritable from cell to cell.

Flashback

An intrusive memory of a traumatic event. Flashbacks are triggered instantly and suddenly. The terror reaction is dormant in the body, which is in a constant state of alert. An odour, sound or other sensory information may suffice to trigger the alarm. With violent force, it casts the person back to the time and reality when the dangerous events took place. Emotional parts in a person with trauma-related dissociation often have powerful flashbacks and feel as if earlier traumatic events were taking place here and now.

Fragmentation

Division or separation. In psychology, the word 'fragmentation' describes division of a person into two or more dissociative parts, which then coexist inside that person. Fragmentation is a symptom of structural dissociation.

Freeze

The state we immediately get into in an acutely dangerous situation when something threatens us. Freezing is often confused with lying down and playing dead. When we freeze, we are absolutely still, take in every impression and decide which of the three strategies — escaping, fighting or playing dead — affords the greatest chance of survival and will minimise our suffering. It is a lightning-fast, unconscious bodily process.

Hippocampus

Region of the brain that receives impulses from sensory organs and helps us to store memories. The hippocampus, part of the limbic system, acts as a kind of switching station that links incomplete memories to form a whole. The hippocampus and amygdala work closely together. In stress, PTSD and severe dissociation, the hippocampus may shrink, making it difficult to remember. However, the area is highly plastic and can regain its normal size.

ICD system

ICD is the World Health Organization's (WHO) international statistical classification system with diagnostic codes that group diseases and causes of death to permit comprehensive statistical compilations and analyses. The latest version, ICD-11 (the 11th revision, 2019) is now a work in progress for every country to incorporate in its health care system.

Integrative psychotherapy

Here, the therapist uses several different methods to create the best possible means of development for the person being treated. The starting point is that humans are versatile and complex beings.

Lithium

Substance often used as medication for bipolar disorder, for example.

MBCT

See MBSR.

MBSR

Mindfulness-based stress reduction, a method developed by Jon Kabat-Zinn (US) and others. The method consists of exercises such as body scanning, mindful movements and meditation. Mindfulness-based cognitive therapy (MBCT), is developed from MBSR and also includes cognitive exercises. MBCT was developed by Mark Williams (UK), mainly for people with recurrent depression.

Mindfulness

The ability to be in touch with the present, which can be developed through an ancient Buddhist method that can be practised to an infinite degree. Mindfulness-based training involves exercising one's senses to make them alert and mindful here and now, without judging oneself. Attention is trained by focusing on bodily sensations, feelings and thoughts.

MRI

Magnetic resonance imaging, a type of medical imaging technique used to form pictures of the anatomy and physiological processes of the body. MRI scanners use strong magnetic fields and radio waves to generate images of the organs in the body, for example to study the brain.

Neglect

Every child must bond to survive. Neglected children are those who are not truly seen by those around them and do not get the affirmation they need — neither the essential attention and understanding, nor help in interpreting their own sensory perceptions or the behaviour of others. Emotional abandonment leads to a 'neglect trauma'. The child's fragmented world fails to grow into one. There is no integration into a cohesive self.

Neuropsychology

A relatively young science in which the relationship between human behaviour and brain function is studied. Neuropsychological research uses images of the brain to examine which areas are active during various states, such as stress and depression, and how meditation affects the workings of the brain.

OSDD

Other specified dissociative disorder, also known as complex PTSD. A person who meets the criteria has a more severe degree of traumatisation than one with PTSD, but does not meet all of the criteria for a diagnosis of DID. The term 'DESNOS' (Disorders of extreme stress not otherwise specified) is also used internationally.

PET

Position emission tomography, a type of scanning that uses small amounts of radioactive materials to evaluate organ functions. PET technique produces a 3-D image of processes in the body and is used to view brain disorders. The information obtained by PET scan, identifying changes at the cellular level, is unique and unavailable with other types of imaging.

Phase-oriented trauma-focused psychotherapy

A therapeutic method for people with severe trauma-related dissociation. The treatment comprises three phases: stabilisation, processing and integration. All three are equally essential for victims to become free from their traumatisation. During the processing phase, the emphasis is on the necessary exposure to traumatic memories. This therapeutic method was developed by Onno van der Hart (Netherlands), Ellert Nijenhuis (Netherlands), Kathy Steele (US) and others.

Phobia

A type of anxiety disorder that hinders normal functioning and involves fear that is irrational, excessive and disproportionate to the situation.

Prefrontal cortex

See Cerebral cortex.

PTSD

Post-traumatic stress disorder, a diagnosis used when people have been traumatised after one or more events that they perceived as overwhelming and life-threatening. Such trauma causes symptoms that people are unable to handle unaided. See Simple PTSD and Complex PTSD.

Rating scale

Based on how people respond to questions, and rate their own symptoms and health. Such self-assessment scales facilitate the therapist's assessment, for example in diagnostics, but are always supplemented with interviews and observation. The questions in a rating scale are based on research on large groups of patients.

Relational mindfulness

Simultaneously relating to others and being actively mindful in the present. Relational mindfulness can be trained in several ways.

Relational psychotherapy

An umbrella term for therapeutic methods aiming to confer the basic security that the person lacks. Early experiences during our first years of life create patterns in us that affect our later relationships. If our patterns have not become secure, we find it difficult to form and maintain close relationships, while we are firmly anchored in a 'self'. In relational psychotherapy, the therapist and patient work together to create this security.

Retraumatisation

Renewed or repeated traumatisation as a result of a new event. This can sometimes aggravate the traumatised person's condition. Unfortunately, the new experience may be caused entirely unnecessarily, for example through excessive exposure of the patient's past trauma by a therapist.

Schizophrenia

A serious psychiatric illness belonging to the psychotic illness group. The perception of being persecuted is often dominant. Delusions are common symptoms. However, schizophrenic patients do not present with different dissociative parts. Although the term 'schizophrenia' has, unfortunately, been used incorrectly for film characters with 'split personality', DID and schizophrenia are thus two completely different types of mental disorder.

Self-compassion

The ability to feel the same compassion for oneself as for other living creatures. We human beings have an innate ability and will to help ourselves and others when someone is having a difficult time, but if we are not used to treating ourselves with understanding and warmth, we criticise and judge ourselves. The capacity for self-compassion can improve with training.

Simple PTSD

The least complicated type of post-traumatic condition. It may occur as a result of one or a few traumatising events. The victim may experience the symptoms as highly troublesome, but simple PTSD is relatively easy to treat. The symptoms usually disappear after a few treatment sessions.

Somatoform dissociation

A diagnosis characterised by the person having physical symptoms with mental causes. Bodily functions are affected, but not in ways that can be explained by organically measurable causes. These seemingly inexplicable difficulties may, for example, involve numbness in the whole or parts of the body, extremely painful urination and temporary inability to hear or see.

Structural dissociation

An umbrella term for the most severe dissociative states, DDNOS and DID. The term is used when dissociative symptoms have created a complex internal pattern in a person whose traumatisation began early in life and has recurred again and again.

Subsystem

Where there is profound splitting in a person's mind, insufficiently integrated subsystems, with various dissociative parts or aspects of the person, have arisen. In one and the same person, there are thus several subsystems or parts who can say *'I want...'* or *'I am...'*. There are not in fact, of course, several individuals in the same body, but the parts themselves have such strong convictions that the outcome is perceived 'selves' that dominate the body at different times. See also ANP and EP.

Suicide risk assessment

A method used by health professionals to try to determine the risk that a person will commit or attempt suicide. Rating scales and interview tools are used in this assessment.

Threat system

Nature has equipped us with reactions that enable us to survive. When we suffer abuse and other unbearable events, the threat system takes over. If, early in life, we face situations that we experience as life-threatening, the threat system becomes hypersensitive. All our senses are then constantly on tenterhooks, and we are ready to defend ourselves at any moment. Vigilance and nervous tension mean that rest and recovery are in short supply.

Time of trauma

The time or period when traumatising events occurred, such as the infant years. Memories from the time can be triggered by, for example, smells, sounds and tastes associated with the event. The traumatised person is instantly cast back to the time of trauma, loses touch with reality here and now and relives the trauma. The fear becomes just as real as if the person were being repeatedly subjected to abuse. Traumatised people may be considered to be living in both the time of trauma and the present. The more severely traumatised they are, the more intense their time confusion.

Trauma

The word originates from Greek and means 'wound' or 'injury'. A medical trauma may be a broken leg caused by an accident. A psychological trauma can occur after a shocking, painful experience. The mind is wounded. An insecure upbringing, characterised by violence and abuse, causes deep wounds. Traumatic memories remain and continue to affect our lives. Trauma in childhood can deeply damage our ability to merge into a unified person. When integration fails, dissociative parts of the personality can be created.

Trauma-focused psychotherapy

See Phase-oriented trauma-focused psychotherapy.

Trauma scripts

Personal trauma narratives.

Traumatisation

If people are involved in events that are so stressful that they cannot cope with their feelings of helplessness or terror, they cannot mentally integrate the experience. This difficulty in embracing reality is at the core of traumatisation. If children suffer painful events at an early age, without getting help in dealing with their own reactions, their risk of traumatisation is elevated. There are various degrees of traumatisation, from PTSD to severe forms of dissociation.

Trigger

Something that invokes memory fragments from traumatic experiences and initiates strong emotional reactions. Without being aware of it, we associate current impressions with what we have known earlier in life. A trigger can come from outside, such as the smell of stale beer, or from inside, in the form of a thought or feeling. The trigger sets off anxiety, rage and other strong feelings that may seem irrelevant in the present.

TRAUMA SCALE

PTSD, Complex PTSD, Minor DID, Major DID

A simplified explanation of various levels of traumatisation:

(Simple) PTSD / Complex PTSD (OSDD) / Minor DID (DDNOS) / Major DID (DID)

|---|

Primary traumatisation   Secondary   Tertiary

A traumatised person is located somewhere along this trauma scale.

PTSD (primary traumatisation) is the mildest degree of damage. If there are deficiencies in basic security during childhood and the attachment pattern becomes insecure, children's vulnerability increases. If they suffer painful events at an early age without receiving help in dealing with their reactions, the risk of traumatisation is elevated. If the events are also recurrent and these children have the misfortune of continuously suffering neglect or abuse, perhaps even at the hands of adults in their immediate vicinity, the risk of complex PTSD (also called OSDD) increases.

Severe trauma-related dissociative disorders affect only people who suffered repeated trauma at an early age. There is no exact research on the age concerned, but it is usually said to be before six to eight years. Experiencing extreme neglect and abuse early in life can lead to extremely complex conditions, known as structural dissociation (secondary or tertiary traumatisation, or DDNOS and DID — also known as minor and major DID — respectively).

Simple PTSD is sometimes called 'Type I trauma' and complex PTSD 'Type II trauma'. In the most recent DSM manual, a subcategory of PTSD has been introduced. There, a few of the dissociative symptoms come to the fore for victims when their various senses and thoughts are stimulated in ways reminiscent of previous traumatic experiences.

GROUP MANUALS

Before a course of trauma-focused psychotherapy starts, the patient's degree of dissociation needs to be identified and diagnosed. There are manuals for patients both with complex PTSD and with dissociative disorders. Some parts of the treatment can be provided in groups.

One group-based manual for complex PTSD was developed by Ethy Dorrepaal, Kathleen Thomaes and Nel Draijer from the Netherlands.

There is also a guide to managing dissociative disorders developed by Suzette Boon, Kathy Steele and Onno van der Hart. This manual, *Coping with Trauma-Related Dissociation: Skills Training for Patients and Therapists*, is intended for group treatment but can also serve as support in individual therapies. The first few chapters explain dissociation very well.

The authors strongly recommend manual users to familiarise themselves with the updated International Society for the Study of Trauma and Dissociation (ISSTD) publication entitled *Guidelines for Treating Dissociative Identity Disorder in Adults*. We understand its message: acquire knowledge, more knowledge and yet more knowledge and experience.

WANT TO READ MORE?

Books

Emerson D, West J. (2015) Trauma-sensitive yoga in therapy: Bringing the body into treatment

Fisher, J. (2017) *Healing the fragmented selves of trauma survivors*

Levine, P. A. (2010) *In an unspoken voice: How the body releases trauma and restores goodness*

Lewis Herman, J. (2007) *Trauma and recovery*

Nijenhuis, E.R.S. (2015) The trinity of trauma: Ignorance, fragility and control: Volume I & II

Nijenhuis, E.R.S. (2017) *The trinity of trauma: Ignorance, fragility, and control: Volume III, Enactive trauma therapy*

Nijenhuis, E.R.S. (2004). *Somatoform dissociation: Phenomena, measurement, and theoretical issues*

Ogden, P. et al (2015) *Sensorimotor Psychotherapy: Interventions for Trauma and Attachment*

Ogden, P, Minton K, Pain, C. (2006) *Trauma and the body: A sensorimotor approach to psychotherapy*

Steele K, Boon S, Van der Hart O. (2011) Treatment manual for groups: Coping with trauma-related dissociation: Skills training for patients and therapists

Steele K, Boon S, Van der Hart O. (2017) Treating trauma-related dissociation: A practical integrative approach

Treleaven D. A, Britton W. (2018) Trauma-sensitive mindfulness: Practices for safe and transformative healing

Van der Hart, O, Nijenhuis, E.R.S, Steele, K. (2006) The haunted self: Structural dissociation and the treatment of chronic traumatization

Research articles

Link to article about fantasy proneness:

Is it Trauma- or Fantasy-based? Comparing dissociative identity disorder, post-traumatic stress disorder, simulators, and controls. Acta Psychiatrica Scandinavica, 1-18. Vissia, E. M., Giesen, M. E., Chalavi, S., Nijenhuis, E. R. S., Draijer, N., Brand, B. L., Reinders, A. A. T. S. (2016).

Link to article about the psychobiology of authentic and simulated dissociative personality states:

https://journals.lww.com/jonmd/Abstract/2016/06000/The_Psychobiology_of_Authentic_and_Simulated.6.aspx

Antje A.T.S. Reinders, Antoon T.M. Willemsen, Eline M. Vissia, Herry P.J. Vos, Johan A. den Boer, & E.R.S. Nijenhuis (2016)

Other articles on the topic by E.R.S Nijenhuis you will find on this link: http://www.enijenhuis.nl/publications

Research article about integrative psychiatry in Psychiatry Today:

https://www.psychiatrictimes.com/integrative-psychiatry/top-down-plus-bottom-integrative-treatments-psychiatry

Research article showing how important positive childhood experiences are for long-term health:

https://m.medicalxpress.com/news/2019-09-kids-trauma-good-neighbors-teachers.html?fbclid=IwAR26kXA2pa1GznzaUFpebDuhbhDfPA2rDVPW_8ObJkxED0ZwPmTnfwkoMOs

Web pages

www.enijenhuis.nl

www.estd.org

www.isst-d.org

www.istss.org

www.nicabm.com

www.thetraumatherapistproject.com/podcast/kathy-steele-mn-cs/

Meditation, compassion & self-compassion

Books

Gilbert, P. (2010) Compassion focused therapy

Goldstein, J, Kornfield, J. (1987) *Seeking the heart of wisdom*

Kabat-Zinn, J. (2004) Wherever you go, there you are: Mindfulness meditation for everyday life

Kabat-Zinn, J. (2005) *Coming to our senses*

Kabat-Zinn, J. (1990) Full catastrophe living

Kornfield, J. (1993) *A path with heart*

Kornfield, J. (2009 *The wise heart*

Neff, K, Germer, C. (2018) The mindful self-compassion workbook: A proven way to accept yourself, build inner strenght, and thrive

Ricard, M. (2010) *Why meditate?*

Teasdale, J, Williams, M.G. et al. (2014) *The mindful way workbook: An 8-week program to free yourself from depression and emotional distress*

Yongey Mingyur Rinpoche (2007) The joy of living: Unlocking the secret & science of happiness

Yongey Mingyur Rinpoche, Swanson E. (2009) Joyful wisdom: Embracing change and finding freedom

Williams, M.G, Teasdale, J, Segal, Z.V, Kabat-Zinn, J. (2007) The mindful way through depression: Freeing yourself from chronic unhappiness

Research links

A free e-book by one famous researcher on self-compassion: *Compassion, bridging practice and science*, Tania Singer and Matthias Bolz:
https://www.goodreads.com/book/show/25411854-compassion-bridging-practice-and-science

Tania Singer on difference between empathy and compassion:
https://vimeo.com/73078925

Tania Singer on Empathy and compassion:
https://www.researchgate.net/publication/265909916_Empathy_and_Compassion

Differential Effects of Attetion_,Compassion-,and Socio-CognitivlyBased Mental Practices on Self-Reports of Mindfulness and Compassion, Lea K.Hildebrandt, Cade McCall, Tania Singer:
https://link.springer.com/article/10.1007/s12671-017-0716-z

Compassion focused theraphy:
https://goo.gl/hDc7rO

Self-compassion in trauma survivors:
https://self-compassion.org/wp-content/uploads/2015/08/Germer.Neff_.Trauma.pdf

CCARE – The Center for Compassion and Altruism Research and Education at Stanford University

https://ccare.stanford.edu/#2

Articles about compassion-meditation

https://scholar.google.se/scholar?q=compassion+meditation&btnG=&hl=sv&as_sdt=0%2C5&as_vis=1

Contenplative research, Alan Wallace

https://www.sbinstitute.com

Informal talk about compassion:

https://vimeo.com/73685698

Neuroscientists and Buddhist agree; counsiousness is everywhere:

https://www.lionsroar.com/christof-koch-unites-buddhist-neuroscience-universal-nature-mind/

Web pages

www.goamra.org

www.karuna-institute.co.uk/index.html

www.metta.org

www.mindandlife.org

www.self-compassion.org

www.springer.com/psychology/cognitive+psychology/journal/12671

www.tergar.org

www.umassmed.edu

FINNS OCKSÅ PÅ SVENSKA

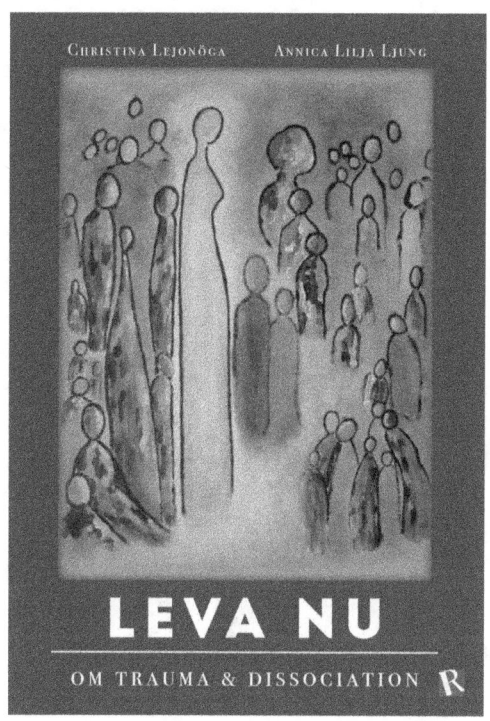

Leva nu : Om trauma & dissociation
Av Christina Lejonöga och Annica Lilja Ljung
Publicerad avRecito Förlag, 2018
Häftad
Antal sidor: 358 st
Vikt: 574 g
Format (b x h): 148 x 210 mm
ISBN: 9789177652250

Available worldwide from
Amazon and all good bookstores

———————

www.mtp.agency

www.facebook.com/mtp.agency

@mtp_agency

www.ingramcontent.com/pod-product-compliance
Lightning Source LLC
LaVergne TN
LVHW012033070526
838202LV00056B/5487